For Elsevier

Commissioning Editor: Fiona Conn
Development Editor: Helen Leng
Project Manager: Nancy Arnott
Senior Designer: Sarah Russell
Illustrator: Oxford Illustrators
Illustration Manager: Gillian Murray

Adams's
Outline of Fractures
Including joint injuries

David L Hamblen
PhD DSc FRCS (Edinburgh, England, Glasgow)

Emeritus Professor of Orthopaedic Surgery,
University of Glasgow
Visiting Professor University of Strathclyde,
Glasgow, UK

A Hamish R W Simpson
MA(Cantab) DM(Oxon) FRCS(Ed & England)

Professor of Orthopaedics and Trauma,
University of Edinburgh

Twelfth edition

CHURCHILL
LIVINGSTONE

ELSEVIER

EDINBURGH LONDON NEW YORK OXFORD PHILADELPHIA ST LOUIS SYDNEY
TORONTO 2007

CHURCHILL
LIVINGSTONE
ELSEVIER

An imprint of Elsevier Limited

© Longman Group UK Limited 1992
© Churchill Livingstone 1998
© 2007, Elsevier Limited. All rights reserved.

First edition 1957	Seventh edition 1978
Second edition 1958	Eighth edition 1983
Third edition 1960	Ninth edition 1987
Fourth edition 1964	Tenth edition 1992
Fifth edition 1968	Eleventh edition 1999
Sixth edition 1972	Twelfth edition 2007

ISBN: 9780443102974
  Reprinted 2008

International edition ISBN: 9780443102981
  Reprinted 2008

British Library Cataloguing in Publication Data
A catalogue record for this book is available from the British Library

Library of Congress Cataloging in Publication Data
A catalog record for this book is available from the Library of Congress

Note
Knowledge and best practice in this field are constantly changing. As new research and experience broaden our knowledge, changes in practice, treatment and drug therapy may become necessary or appropriate. Readers are advised to check the most current information provided (i) on procedures featured or (ii) by the manufacturer of each product to be administered, to verify the recommended dose or formula, the method and duration of administration, and contraindications. It is the responsibility of the practitioner, relying on their own experience and knowledge of the patient, to make diagnoses, to determine dosages and the best treatment for each individual patient, and to take all appropriate safety precautions. To the fullest extent of the law, neither the publisher nor the authors assume any liability for any injury and/or damage to persons or property arising out or related to any use of the material contained in this book.

The Publisher

Printed in China

Preface

The invitation to produce a new edition of such a well-established textbook as *Outline of Fractures* presented a considerable challenge. The attractions to accept were that the new 12th edition would appear 50 years after John Crawford Adams published the first edition of his book and that his wise guidance was still available to us in its preparation. The science and technology of the management of injuries of the musculoskeletal system has changed dramatically over this time period. Even in the 8 years since the last edition there has been a major shift to a more aggressive surgical approach for the treatment of some common fractures previously managed by conservative methods. This change has been driven as much by health economics and patient demand, as by improved long-term outcomes, and we continue to describe both radical and conservative solutions, where appropriate.

The changes to the content and format also reflect changes in the potential readership since the book, that was once aimed primarily at the medical student, is now used by a broad range of health professionals, including basic surgical trainees. We have not attempted to produce a volume aimed at the specialist orthopaedic surgeon, although much of the content goes beyond the needs of the student or basic practitioner. Some of this additional information was previously presented in a smaller size of print, but in this edition all text has been changed to a standard font format. It is hoped that this will allow the reader the opportunity to study selected topics in greater depth if their interests demand it. The detailed references to other literature have also been removed since these are inevitably becoming out of date by the time of publication. The easy availability of this information on the Internet through links to orthopaedic and scientific literature websites provides a far more satisfactory alternative. We have added one new chapter to address the important topic of osteoporosis and its association with fragility fractures in the elderly. This is now recognised as a major health problem with a world-wide impact, resulting from the increased longevity in ageing populations.

Many of the illustrations have been updated to reflect current treatment trends, but the anatomical classification of injuries has been retained and enhanced. We feel that this provides a more readily understandable basis for the general reader in preference to the more complex treatment-based classifications used by the specialist surgeon. The future direction of fracture treatment is difficult to predict, but some of the newer techniques resulting from developments in cell biology and molecular genetics that allow local stimulation of bone healing have been included.

It is hoped that the book will continue to provide a sound basis for the management of musculoskeletal injuries, based on an amalgam of established traditional conservative methods and safe surgical techniques with proven results.

David L Hamblen
A Hamish R W Simpson

Note by
John Crawford Adams

Fifty years ago, as a young orthopaedic and trauma surgeon at St. Mary's Hospital in London, I developed a keen interest in teaching. Finding that students showed interest in what I taught, I resolved to set down, in an easily read form, the elements of orthopaedic surgery and of fracture management. The material was to be in two slim volumes, and there would be a heavy emphasis on the provision of numerous illustrations of high quality. Although the books would be primarily for the benefit of undergraduate students, they might also be useful for general practitioners and physiotherapists, and even for lawyers. Mr Charles Macmillan of Edinburgh, an enterprising publisher with a prestigious bookshop in Teviot Place, undertook to publish the books. The first of the two books, *Outline of Orthopaedics*, was published in 1956, and was followed in 1957 by the companion volume, *Outline of Fractures*. The books proved popular with medical students and physiotherapists, both in the UK and abroad, and updated editions were called for every few years. By 1990 the task of keeping the texts up to date was proving difficult for me, an ageing author, and I was fortunate that Professor David Hamblen, then Professor of Orthopaedic Surgery in the University of Glasgow, was willing to come to my assistance to help transform the books for the needs of the modern world. But still events move on, and the time has come for me to bow out and to welcome Professor Hamish Simpson, of the University of Edinburgh, to assist Professor Hamblen with the task of once again bringing the books – starting with *Outline of Fractures* – right up to date. In doing so, I thank all those students – many now mature doctors – for their interest in using the books to gain an insight into the fascinating subject of orthopaedic surgery.

John Crawford Adams

Acknowledgements

The authors wish to acknowledge the assistance of a number of colleagues in the preparation of the new edition of this well established text. In particular, we wish to thank the original author, John Crawford Adams, whose inspiration and enthusiasm produced the original volume and steered it through eleven further editions. The success it has enjoyed is a tribute to his writing skills and we were fortunate to have been able to seek his advice, when required.

A large number of additional illustrations have been added to reflect the changes in the diagnosis and treatment of injuries. We thank Dr Nigel Raby of the Western Infirmary, Glasgow, for providing us with the new images of radiographs, CT and MR scans included in many of the chapters.

Mr David Allan, the Director of the Scottish Spinal Injury Centre, and his staff and patients are thanked for providing us with advice and the illustrations used in the chapters on spinal injury and paraplegia.

We are grateful to Dr Robin Reid, Western Infirmary, Glasgow, for providing the images of pathological fractures resulting from primary and secondary bone tumours.

Thanks are also due to Helen Leng, Sarah Russell, Nancy Arnott, and the staff at Elsevier for all their help and encouragement in the production of this new edition.

Our respective secretaries Catherine Davidson and Linda Digance have played a key role in the typing of the manuscript and their efforts are very much appreciated.

Finally, we record our appreciation of the support and forbearance of our wives and families during the time devoted to the writing of the book.

Contents

Introduction

The treatment of fractures on a precise scientific basis has been possible only since adequate radiographic techniques became available. Although Roentgen announced his discovery of X-rays in 1895, several years elapsed before the necessary apparatus was developed for clinical use. So it may be said that modern fracture treatment began to develop at about the beginning of the present century. Before that time surgeons had to rely entirely upon a knowledge of dissected specimens and upon clinical evidence in determining the nature of the injury. It is evident, therefore, that they must have worked largely 'in the dark'.

It was at about the beginning of the century, too, that surgeons began to think more in terms of open operations in the treatment of difficult fractures. Antiseptic surgery (introduced by Lister in 1867) and its offspring aseptic surgery were relatively recent innovations, and before their introduction open operations upon bone were virtually prohibited by the risk of infection.

Even when the advantages of an aseptic technique and of radiography became available, operative fracture surgery was still severely handicapped by the lack of inert metals with which to fix the bones in apposition. Internal appliances of iron, mild steel or silver corroded and partly dissolved away in the tissues, causing a local reaction which often hindered union. This problem was not overcome until the period between the first and second world wars, when metallurgists developed alloys that could remain indefinitely in the tissues without corrosion.

PRESENT TRENDS

In post-war years the trend in fracture treatment has been towards the exercise of sound judgement and common sense rather than a slavish adherence to rigid precepts. No longer is it accepted automatically that because the bone fragments are not in exact apposition manipulation must be carried out: some fractures do not require reduction. Likewise it is no longer held that because a bone is fractured it must necessarily be rigidly immobilised until the fragments are united: some fractures do not need immobilisation. But above all has come the realisation that in the treatment of a fracture it is not the bone alone that matters. Attention must be paid to the soft tissues, and especially to the muscles, whose function must be preserved by active use within the limits imposed by necessary splintage, and redeveloped by graduated activity when the splintage is removed.

The second half of the twentieth century saw dramatic changes in the technology available to assist clinicians in the diagnosis and treatment of all types of musculo-skeletal injury. These allowed a shift to the more frequent use of internal fixation, as an alternative to splintage or traction, for the management

Introduction

of limb bone fractures. This move away from conservative methods was led by the Swiss AO (Arbeitsgemeinshaft für Osteosynthesefragen) fixation group, who first published their new techniques in 1965. These depended on the development of new designs of implants and the instruments to insert them, using advanced engineering methods. Their philosophy of compression fixation also embraced a new biological concept of primary bone healing, instead of by secondary callus formation. These ideas and innovations have been modified and refined by others, particularly in the field of intramedullary nail fixation. The result is that the surgeon of today is faced with an enormous range of bone fixation systems, many of which require specialised training for their safe use. In turn, this has stimulated more educational activity, including 'hands-on' courses, where students learn to apply the techniques to simulated fractures in synthetic bones. Certainly without this training and experience under supervision, surgeons should not attempt to use these complicated technologies.

Another development, in response to the increasing number of open fractures and war injuries, has been the improved designs of external fixator. These permit stabilization of the bone fragments by the insertion of percutaneous pins, which are then attached to a rigid external frame. The method has the advantages of allowing adjustment of the fracture position, as well as permitting reconstructive procedures on the soft tissues.

During the same period methods of conservative treatment have also advanced with the introduction of improved lightweight splinting materials and better designs of splint. These, in combination with the use of functional cast bracing, now allow much earlier mobilization of the patient than was customary in the past. There is now clear evidence that earlier movement of limbs, with both fractures and soft tissue injuries, will promote healing and speed rehabilitation.

These advances in treatment methods could not have occurred without parallel developments in the techniques of bone and soft tissue imaging. The introduction of computerised tomography (CT) radiographic scanning and magnetic resonance imaging (MRI) has revolutionised the way we can look at fractures and joint injuries. The ability to view images in any of three planes, and even in three dimensions, allows better diagnosis and treatment planning for the more complex or multiple injuries. Advances in optical technology have also allowed arthroscopy to be performed on all but the smallest joints, with the ability to repair joint structures, including articular cartilage.

All these new technologies are expensive and many are not available to those working outwith major trauma centres in the developed world. The choice of the best treatment for any patient will depend on their availability and the experience of the surgeon in their use. It has to be acknowledged that there is often more than one way of treating a fracture successfully, and with certain fractures there must always be a divergence of opinion on what is the best method. Some surgeons will always tend towards a conservative approach, whereas others will turn more readily to operative methods. In this book we have tried to strike a fair balance by including both conservative and operative methods for the treatment of individual injuries, where they offer the possibility of an equally successful outcome for the patient.

Pathology of fractures and fracture healing | 1

A fracture may be a complete break in the continuity of a bone or, occasionally, it may be an incomplete break.

CLASSIFICATION

Fractures may be subdivided, according to their aetiology, into four groups:

1. fractures caused solely by sudden injury
2. fragility fractures.
3. fatigue or stress fractures
4. pathological fractures

Fractures caused solely by sudden injury. These fractures form by far the largest group. They occur through bone that was previously free from disease. Such a fracture may be caused by *direct violence*—as when a metatarsal bone is fractured by a heavy weight dropped on the foot; or by *indirect violence* transmitted along the bone—as when the head of the radius is fractured in a fall on the outstretched hand, or the clavicle in a fall on the shoulder.

Fragility fractures. This term is now used for the increasing number of fractures associated with a generalised bone weakness resulting from the condition of osteoporosis, seen most commonly in elderly patients. These fractures and their management are described more fully in Chapter 6, page 79.

So great is the preponderance of these groups over the other two, the term 'fracture', if unqualified, is generally taken to signify these type of injuries.

Fatigue fractures. Fatigue or stress fractures occur not from a single violent injury but from oft-repeated stress, and commonly occur in athletes or new military recruits. They occur when the rate of microdamage exceeds the rate of repair. In these circumstances, the microdamage accumulates and progresses to a complete fracture across the full width of the bones. They have been likened to the fractures that occur in certain metals when 'fatigued' by repeated stress. With few exceptions, fatigue or stress fractures are confined to the bones of the lower limb. The great majority occurs in the metatarsals, but other well recognised sites are the shaft of the fibula, the shaft of the tibia and the neck of the femur.

Pathological fractures. The term 'pathological' is applied to a fracture through a bone already weakened by disease. A fracture is pathological if it is created by a level of force that would not have resulted in a fracture in a healthy bone. Often the bone gives way from trivial violence, or even spontaneously. The causes of pathological fractures will be considered later (p. 16).

Fig. 1.1 [A] Closed or simple fracture. There is no communication between the fractured bone and the body surface. [B] Open or compound fracture. There is a wound leading down to the site of fracture. Organisms may gain access through the wound and infect the bone.

CLOSED AND OPEN FRACTURES

A fracture is closed or simple when there is no communication between the site of fracture and the exterior of the body (Fig. 1.1A). A fracture is open or compound when there is a wound of the skin surface (intestinal mucosa, cranial sinuses, or pleural space) leading down to the site of fracture (Fig. 1.1B). It must be stressed that the presence of a wound of the skin in association with a fracture does not necessarily mean that the fracture is an open fracture: it is classed as open or compound only when a direct communication exists between the body surface and the fractured bone ends. The communication may be through an open wound, but it may be no more than a puncture wound or even an area of bruised and devitalised skin.

The distinction between closed and open fractures is important, because an open fracture is liable to be contaminated by organisms introduced from without and may therefore become infected, whereas infection of a closed fracture is exceedingly rare unless it has been operated upon.

PATTERNS OF FRACTURE

Fractures are often designated by descriptive terms denoting the shape or pattern of the fracture surfaces as seen on radiographs (Fig. 1.2). The following terms are in general use: transverse fractures; oblique fractures; spiral fractures; comminuted fractures (with more than two fragments); compression or crush fractures; greenstick fractures (incomplete breaks occurring only in the resilient bones of children). Impacted fractures are those in which the bone fragments are driven so firmly together that they become interlocked and there is no movement between them.

Fig. 1.2 Common patterns of fracture. A Transverse fracture; B oblique fracture; C spiral fracture; D comminuted fracture; E compression fracture; F greenstick fractures.

The pattern of fracture is of more than academic interest. It may indicate the nature of the causative violence and may thus give a clue to the easiest method of reduction. For instance, a fracture occurring transversely through a long bone has almost certainly been caused by an angulation force rather than a twisting force, whereas a spiral fracture has equally surely been caused by a twisting force.[1]

The pattern of fracture also gives an indication of the likely stability of the fragments. Thus a transverse fracture is unlikely to become redisplaced after reduction, whereas an oblique or spiral fracture is prone to redisplacement unless projecting spikes of bone can be locked into notches in the opposing surface (Fig. 1.3). A compression fracture (Fig. 1.2, diagram E) does not always lend itself well to anatomical reduction, because the spongy bone substance

[1] In its behaviour to violence an adult long bone may be compared with a stick of chalk. A simple experiment will show that the chalk is broken transversely if an angulatory force is applied, whereas it breaks spirally if a twisting force is used.

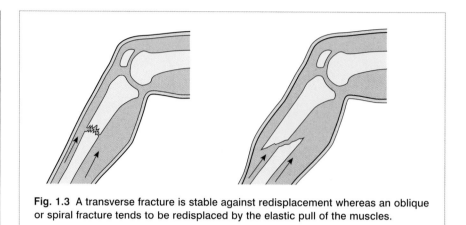

Fig. 1.3 A transverse fracture is stable against redisplacement whereas an oblique or spiral fracture tends to be redisplaced by the elastic pull of the muscles.

may be crushed and compressed and cannot be restored fully to its original trabecular form.

Greenstick fractures are peculiar to children, whose bones, especially before the age of 10 years, are springy and resilient like the branches of a young tree. Bone of this type can be 'crumpled' like a concertina by a longitudinal compression force (Fig. 1.4A). An angulation force tends to bend the bone at one cortex and to buckle or break it at the other, thus producing an incomplete fracture (buckle fracture or torus fracture) (Fig. 1.4B). Although with severe violence children's bones often suffer complete fracture, incomplete fractures of the greenstick type are more common, especially in young children.

Fig. 1.4 Radiographs of typical greenstick fractures in children. The fractures in A were caused by a longitudinal compression force and those in B by an angulation force.

HEALING OF FRACTURES

A fracture begins to heal as soon as the bone is broken and, provided the conditions are favourable, healing proceeds through several stages until the bone is consolidated (Fig. 1.5).

The histological features of fracture repair at various intervals after injury were well described by Ham and Harris in 1956. Their description applied mainly to rib fractures in the rabbit, but the evidence suggests that the repair process is similar in humans, at any rate when the conditions are comparable. Nevertheless, it must be appreciated that the pattern of healing is not constant for all bones and in all circumstances. The repair of a tubular bone shows striking differences from the repair of a cancellous bone, and the pattern of healing in a given bone is probably influenced by such factors as the rigidity of fixation of the fragments and the closeness of their coaptation.

REPAIR OF TUBULAR BONE

For purposes of simplicity the process of healing of a fractured tubular bone may be considered as occurring in five stages:

1. stage of haematoma
2. stage of subperiosteal and endosteal cellular proliferation
3. stage of callus
4. stage of consolidation
5. remodelling.

It must be emphasised, however, that these stages are not sharply demarcated and that two or more stages of healing may be seen at the same time in different parts of the bone. The process of healing of a tubular bone is illustrated in Figure 1.5.

Stage of haematoma (Fig. 1.5A)
When a bone is fractured, blood seeps out through torn vessels and forms a haematoma between and around the fracture surfaces. The haematoma is largely contained by the surrounding periosteum, which may be stripped up or torn from the bone ends to a variable extent. Where the periosteum is torn, the haematoma is extravasated into the soft tissues, being contained ultimately by muscles, fascia and skin.

The fracture inevitably divides most of the capillaries that run longitudinally in the compact bone, and the ring of bone immediately adjacent to each side of the fracture becomes ischaemic over a variable length, usually a few millimetres. Deprived of their blood supply, the osteocytes near the fracture surfaces die. The blood contributes various growth factors which help to attract cells into the fracture site.

Stage of subperiosteal and endosteal cellular proliferation (Fig. 1.5B)
The most prominent feature in the early stages of repair is proliferation of cells from the deep surface of the periosteum close to the fracture. These cells are the precursors of osteoblasts, which will later lay down the intercellular substance. They form a collar of active tissue that surrounds each fragment and grows out towards the other fragment.

Pathology of fractures and fracture healing

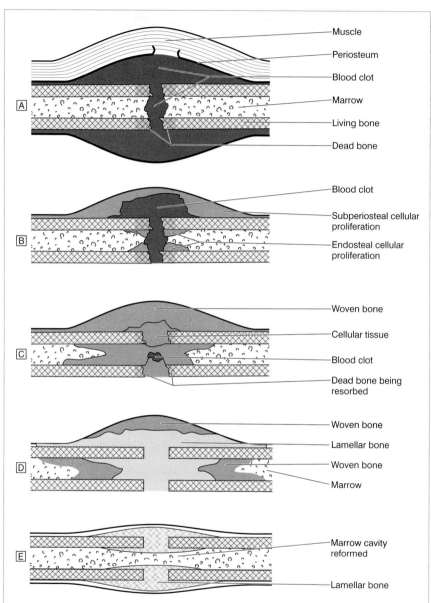

Fig. 1.5 Stages in the healing of a fracture. A Stage of haematoma, with necrosis of bone immediately adjacent to the fracture. B Stage of subperiosteal and endosteal cellular proliferation. The cellular tissue, which may contain islands of cartilage, pushes forward from each side of the fracture at the expense of the blood clot. C Stage of callus. The proliferating cells give rise to osteoblasts, which lay down intercellular substance; this becomes calcified, to form woven bone or callus. D Stage of consolidation. Osteoblasts continue the process of repair, laying down lamellar bone at the expense of the woven bone. E Remodelling. Bone is strengthened in the lines of stress and resorbed elsewhere. The bone is thus restored more or less to its original form.

Simultaneously with the subperiosteal proliferation there is cellular activity within the medullary canal, where the proliferating cells appear to be derived from the endosteum and from the marrow tissue of each fragment. This tissue, too, grows forward to meet and blend with similar tissue growing from the other fragment.

Within the cellular tissue that grows forward outside and inside the bone to bridge the fracture, there may be seen islands of cartilage. The cartilage is variable in amount: sometimes it is profuse but it may be absent. Evidently it is not an essential element in the process of healing.

Stage of callus (Fig. 1.5C)

As the cellular tissue that has grown out from each fragment matures, the basic cells give rise to osteoblasts and, in places, to chondroblasts, which form the cartilage already referred to. The osteoblasts lay down an intercellular matrix of collagen and polysaccharide, which soon becomes impregnated with calcium salts to form the immature bone or osteoid of fracture callus. This, from its texture, has been termed 'woven' bone (Fig. 1.6). The formation of this

Fig. 1.6 Section showing a healing fracture of human rib 3 weeks after injury. The fracture is seen in the lower part of the section. In the limited area shown, the original bone fragments are dead (db), as indicated by the empty lacunae. Between the fragments is nothing more than old blood clot (bc): union is occurring mainly around the periphery of the fracture. Next to the bone (near bottom left) is a thin layer of woven bone (wb). Above this, near the middle of the section, is young fibrous tissue (ft), bounded above by the old periosteum (pm). Outside this is a thicker layer of typical woven bone, and outside this again is the new periosteum. (Haematoxylin and eosin, × 40.)

Pathology of fractures and fracture healing

bridge of woven bone imparts rigidity to the fracture, and when the injured bone is a superficial one the callus may be felt as a hard mass surrounding the fracture. The mass of callus or woven bone is also visible in radiographs and gives the first radiological indication that the fracture is uniting.

Stage of consolidation (Fig. 1.5D)
The woven bone that forms the primary callus is gradually transformed by the combined activity of osteoclasts and osteoblasts into more mature bone with a typical lamellar structure.

Stage of remodelling (Fig. 1.5E)
When union is complete the newly formed bone often forms a bulbous collar, which surrounds the bone and obliterates the medullary canal (Fig. 1.5, diagram D). The size of the mass varies from case to case. It tends to be large when there has been much periosteal stripping, when the fracture haematoma has been large, and when there is marked displacement of the fragments. It is usually small when the bone fragments are in exact anatomical apposition, and especially when the fragments are rigidly fixed in close apposition by a metal plate with screws or by an intramedullary nail. Callus is usually profuse in children, because the periosteum is easily stripped from the bone by extravasated blood, allowing bone to form beneath it.

In the months that follow union, the bone is gradually strengthened along the lines of stress at the expense of the surplus bone outside the lines of stress, which is slowly removed. This process of remodelling is going on constantly, but inconspicuously, in every bone throughout life, but it becomes especially obvious after a fracture.

In children, remodelling after a fracture is usually so perfect that eventually the site of the fracture becomes indistinguishable on radiographs (Fig. 1.7). In adults, remodelling generally falls short of this ideal, and the site of a fracture is usually permanently marked by an area of thickening or sclerosis.

REPAIR OF CANCELLOUS BONE

Healing of a fractured cancellous bone follows a different pattern from that of a tubular bone. Because the bone is of a uniform spongy texture and has no medullary canal, there is, relatively, a much broader area of contact between the fragments than in the case of a tubular bone, and the open meshwork of trabeculae allows easier penetration by bone-forming tissue. Union can occur directly between the bone surfaces and it does not have to take place through the medium of external callus, as in a tubular bone.

The first stage of healing is the formation of a haematoma, into which new blood vessels and proliferating osteogenic cells from the fracture surfaces penetrate until they meet and fuse with similar tissue growing out from the opposing fragment. Osteoblasts then lay down the intercellular matrix, which becomes calcified to form woven bone.

Fig. 1.7 Remodelling after a fracture of the femur in a child of 7 years. The interval between the two radiographs was just over 1 year.

Origin and activation of bone-forming cells

The foregoing is no more than a basic sketch of the processes concerned in the repair of a fracture. There has been much research into the complex biological processes by which repair is initiated and carried through to its completion, but many of the details are still not fully understood.

The actual laying down of bone is clearly a function of osteoblasts, but there has been much discussion on where they come from, and particularly on what stimulates them to activity. It seems clear that the deep surface of the periosteum contains 'resting' osteoblasts which are capable of activation and proliferation under the appropriate stimulus. Similar 'resting' osteoblasts are believed to exist in the endosteum, the thin layer that lines the medullary canal of the long bones.

Pathology of fractures and fracture healing

Whatever may be the contribution of these sources, there is also convincing evidence that osteoblasts may be newly formed in the bone marrow from progenitor, or precursor, cells, i.e. stem cells. The mechanism by which these cells are stimulated to differentiate into osteoblasts is believed to be a chemical one, dependent upon a specific substance liberated in the region of the fracture, possibly by necrotic cells. More recent work suggests that a variety of different types of cell (chondroblasts, osteoprogenitor cells, platelets) can produce specific mitogenic bone growth factors which may be important in stimulating the repair process.

It is thought also that endocrine factors may play a part, as it has been shown that systemic effects of an injury may lead to an increased release of parathyroid hormone into the circulation, and that this may be a factor in the promotion of increased periosteal and endosteal cell proliferation.

The work of Trueta (1963), embodying studies with the electron microscope, emphasised the important part played by the small blood vessels—capillaries and sinusoids—in the repair of a fracture. He concluded that new blood vessels are attracted centripetally towards the fracture from the surrounding area, possibly under the stimulus of a chemical inductor substance liberated by sick or dead osteocytes in the ischaemic bone adjacent to the fracture. He showed that the endothelial cells that line these new blood vessels can divide to form migratory 'intermediate' cells that are the precursors of osteoblasts. Moreover, he found that these osteoblasts retain a direct cytoplasmic connection, through their filamentous processes, with the ancestral endothelial cells, whence presumably they derive their blood-borne nutriment. When these osteoblasts finally surround themselves with intercellular substance and become osteocytes, locked each in its own lacuna, the fine cytoplasmic filaments still persist within the canaliculi of the Haversian systems. Trueta claimed further that the small blood vessels of bone are important agents in bone resorption, a fundamental part of the process of remodelling. The most active agents of bone resorption, the multinucleated osteoclasts, are formed from a separate line of bone marrow stem cells and are not, as was once thought, derived from osteoblasts.

RATE OF UNION

The time taken for a fracture to unite is so variable that hard and fast rules cannot be laid down. In young children union is nearly always rapid, callus often being visible radiologically within 2 weeks and the bone being consolidated in 4 or 6 weeks (Fig. 1.8). In older children, union occurs a little less rapidly. When adult life is reached, age has a far smaller effect upon the rate of union.

In adults the time usually required for consolidation of a fractured long bone, in favourable conditions, is about 3 months, though in many cases it extends to 4 or even 5 months, especially in the case of a large bone such as the femur. In general, union tends to occur rather more rapidly in the slender bones of the upper limbs than in the large weight-bearing bones of the lower limbs.

Fractures through cancellous bone unite in a somewhat shorter time than fractures through hard cortical bone.

Fig. 1.8 A Radiographs illustrating the speed with which fractures unite in young children. Initial radiographs of a fractured femur in a child of 8 years.
B Three weeks later, showing advanced callus formation. A similar fracture in an adult would be expected to take at least 3 months to reach the same stage of union.

Factors that influence the speed of union

Several factors, apart from the age of the patient and the type of bone (cortical or cancellous), may influence the speed of union. Favourable factors are a plentiful supply of blood to the bone fragments and, important in some fractures, immobility. Conversely, union may be hindered or even prevented by impairment of the blood supply even to one of the fragments, or by movement between the fragments. That is not to say, however, that movement is always harmful: many fractures unite readily despite almost constant movement between the fragments—for instance, fractures of the ribs, clavicle or shaft of the femur. In these instances movement is angulatory and does not damage the flexible granulations that bridge the fracture from an early stage. Movement that is harmful is usually rotatory or shearing movement, which may sever the delicate capillaries in the bridging tissue: such movement is liable to occur particularly in fractures of the forearm bones, scaphoid bone and the neck of the femur, if the fragments are not perfectly immobilised. Other factors that may hinder union are infection of the bone, interposition of soft tissue, or involvement of the bone by a tumour. A fracture within a joint may be more liable than most other fractures to non-union, possibly because the presence of synovial fluid about the site of fracture hinders the formation of granulation tissue across the fracture gap. These matters are considered further in the section on delayed union and non-union of fractures (p. 54).

FATIGUE OR STRESS FRACTURES

Fatigue fractures in metal are well known to engineers. In consequence of repeated stress there is a gradual rearrangement of molecular structure which weakens the metal and permits a crack to occur. A similar mechanism of crack accumulation is thought to occur in bone, although the composite nature of bone makes it more resistant to propagation of the cracks. The analogy between fatigue fractures in metal and those seen clinically in humans is apt so far as the predisposing cause is concerned. In most cases of fatigue fracture of bone there is a history of oft-repeated minor stresses preceding the onset of pain: prolonged walking or marching in the case of fractures of the metatarsal bones, and repeated running or dancing in the case of fractures of the fibula or tibia. These three bones, metatarsal, fibula and tibia are the most common sites of fatigue fracture in that order, but the femur and occasionally other bones may be affected.

The great difference between a fatigue fracture and an ordinary 'traumatic' fracture is that there is no single specific causative injury in cases of fatigue fracture. The onset of pain in the affected bone is gradual or insidious, seldom abrupt. The pain is increased by continued activity and relieved by rest.

A B

Fig. 1.9 Fatigue or stress fracture of the second metatarsal bone, often termed a march fracture. This is the most common site for fatigue fractures. In the first radiograph A, taken soon after the onset of symptoms, the fracture is hardly visible: it can just be seen as a hairline crack (arrow). Two weeks later B the radiograph is much more striking, the fracture now being surrounded by a mass of callus.

Fig. 1.10 Fatigue fracture of lower end of tibia.

Examination reveals well-marked local tenderness over the affected bone. Soon afterwards there is swelling, with perhaps some local thickening, over the site of fracture. It is important to remember that radiologically nothing abnormal may be seen at first: it is only after 2–4 weeks that radiographic changes appear (Figs 1.9 & 1.10). Even then the fracture itself may show only as a faint hairline crack, usually more or less transverse in direction: only rarely is there any displacement of the fragments. More striking than the fracture is the zone of callus that surrounds it. Faint at first—seen only as a haze near the bone—this new bone may eventually form a dense fusiform mass about the site of fracture (Fig. 1.9). It has occasionally been mistaken for a bone sarcoma, an error that should not occur if the features of fatigue fracture are properly understood.

PATHOLOGICAL FRACTURES

A pathological fracture occurs through a bone that is already weakened by disease. Often the bone gives way from trivial violence, or even spontaneously. In many cases the patient, when directly questioned, will admit to having suffered pain or discomfort in the region of the affected bone for some time before the fracture. The underlying disease of the bone may be local and circumscribed, or it may be a generalised disorder affecting several bones or the whole skeleton.

Table 1.1 The more important causes of pathological fracture

Local disease of bone
Infections
Pyogenic osteomyelitis (usually in chronic form)
Benign tumours
Chondroma (enchondroma)
Giant-cell tumour (osteoclastoma)
Haemangioma (spine)
Malignant tumours
Osteosarcoma (osteogenic sarcoma)
Ewing's tumour
Solitary myeloma
Metastatic carcinoma (especially from lung, breast, prostate, thyroid or kidney)
Metastatic sarcoma (from primary in another bone)
Miscellaneous
Simple bone cyst
Monostotic fibrous dysplasia
Eosinophilic granuloma
Bone atrophy in paralytic conditions such as poliomyelitis
Tabes dorsalis
Osteonecrosis after irradiation
General affections of the skeleton
Congenital disorders
Osteogenesis imperfecta (fragilitas ossium)
Diffuse rarefaction of bone
Osteoporosis
Parathyroid osteodystrophy
Cushing's syndrome
Infantile rickets
Coeliac (gluten-induced) rickets
Uraemic osteodystrophy (renal rickets)
Cystinosis (renal tubular rickets; Fanconi syndrome)
Nutritional osteomalacia
Idiopathic steatorrhoea
Disseminated tumours
Multiple myeloma (myelomatosis)
Diffuse metastatic carcinoma
Miscellaneous
Paget's disease (osteitis deformans)
Polyostotic fibrous dysplasia
Gaucher's disease
Hand-Schüller-Christian disease

Fig. 1.11 Examples of pathological fractures. Ⓐ Fracture through a bone cyst in the radius. Ⓑ Fracture through a tibia affected by Paget's disease (osteitis deformans). Ⓒ Fracture at the site of a carcinomatous metastasis in the upper half of the femoral shaft.

Causes

The causes of pathological fractures are shown in Table 1.1 and illustrative radiographs are shown in Figures 1.11–1.13. When a local or circumscribed lesion of bone is responsible, the most common cause is metastatic carcinoma, usually from the lung, breast, prostate, thyroid or kidney. Such fractures occur most frequently in the vertebral bodies (especially of the thoracic or lumbar region) (Fig. 1.12B), in the proximal half of the femoral shaft (Fig. 1.11C) and in the proximal half of the humerus, but no bone is immune. Another common cause is a bone cyst, usually in a long bone (Fig. 1.11A). In cases of pathological fracture from diffuse or generalised affections of the skeleton, the most common cause is osteoporosis, and the bones most often affected are the thoracic or lumbar vertebral bodies (Fig. 1.12A), the neck or trochanteric region of the femur, and the lower end of the radius (see Chapter 6). Another common cause is Paget's disease of bone (osteitis deformans), with fracture usually of the shaft of the tibia or femur (Fig. 1.11B).

Fig. 1.12 Further examples of pathological fractures. [A] Vertebral fractures from generalised osteoporosis. Note the partial collapse of several vertebral bodies, with marked ballooning of the discs at the expense of the vertebral end plates. [B] Vertebral fracture from carcinomatous metastasis. A single vertebral body is affected.

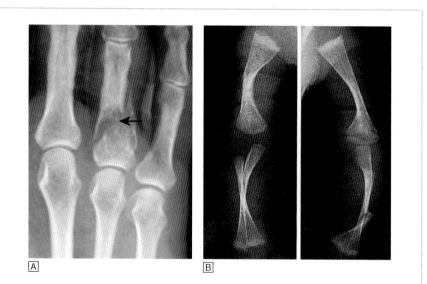

Fig. 1.13 [A] Pathological fracture through a benign chondroma in the proximal phalanx of a finger (arrow). [B] Recent and old fractures of the bones of the upper limbs in an infant with osteogenesis imperfecta (fragilitas ossium).

Will the fracture unite?

Whether or not a pathological fracture will unite depends largely upon the nature of the underlying disorder of the bone. When this is a generalised affection such as osteogenesis imperfecta, Paget's disease (osteitis deformans), or one of the diffuse rarefying diseases of bone (Table 1.1), the fracture may be expected to unite, often in about the usual time but sometimes more slowly than usual. A fracture at the site of a bone cyst or benign tumour will also generally unite, but there may be some delay. On the other hand, in fractures through a bone weakened by infection, union is often seriously delayed or may fail altogether, unless the infection is eradicated. Fractures through the site of a malignant tumour often remain ununited, but union may sometimes occur after treatment.

2 | Clinical and radiological features of fractures

The presence of a fracture can nearly always be inferred from the history and the clinical findings alone, but radiographs are necessary to establish its precise nature.

HISTORY

The statement that a patient is unable to stand or walk after an injury, or use the injured part, must always arouse suspicion of a fracture. The immediate appearance of deformity in a limb bone is clearly diagnostic of fracture. A history of visible bruising, appearing a day or so after an accident, is also suggestive. In many cases, however, the history does not provide reliable evidence on which to distinguish between a fracture and a simple strain or contusion.

Although in most fractures there is a distinct history of injury, it should be remembered that in cases of fatigue fracture and of pathological fracture there may be a spontaneous onset of pain and disability without any causative injury. In some cases of malicious injury to a baby, an accurate account of any incident is deliberately withheld.

Commonly missed fractures
The doctor is sometimes misled into believing that no fracture exists by the fact that the patient has retained the use of the painful limb. In certain cases reasonable function is often preserved despite a fracture. The types of fracture that may be overlooked in this way include impacted fractures, fatigue fractures, fractures of small bones especially in the wrist, fractures of the ribs and, in children, minor greenstick fractures. If the common sites of such fractures are borne in mind, mistakes in diagnosis should be avoided:

- **Impacted fractures:** the most common sites are the neck of the humerus, the lower end of the radius, and the neck of the femur.
- **Fatigue fractures:** the most common sites are the second and third metatarsal bones, and the shaft of the tibia or fibula.
- **Fractures of carpal bones:** fractures of the scaphoid bone are particularly liable to be overlooked.
- **Rib fractures:** despite local tenderness and restriction of respiration, rib fractures sometimes go unrecognised.
- **Greenstick fractures:** these are common in the forearm bones of children.

CLINICAL EXAMINATION

The objective signs of fracture are so well known that only a brief summary is required here. The following features, though not in themselves diagnostic, are fairly constant and should always arouse suspicion of a fracture:

- visible or palpable deformity
- local swelling
- visible bruising (ecchymosis) from escape of blood from the fracture surfaces and periosteum
- marked local tenderness over bone
- marked impairment of function.

The following features give unmistakable evidence of fracture, but they should not be deliberately elicited:

- abnormal mobility (that is, demonstrable movement between the fragments)
- crepitus or grating when the injured part is moved.

Clinical evidence of fracture must always be confirmed or refuted by radiographic examination.

ADDITIONAL CLINICAL INVESTIGATIONS

When a diagnosis of fracture has been made, the surgeon should continue the examination to determine the answers to the following four questions:

1. Is there a wound communicating with the fracture?
2. Is there any impairment of the circulation distal to the fracture?
3. Is there any evidence of nerve injury?
4. Is there any evidence of visceral injury?

These facts should always be ascertained before treatment is begun. The presence of a wound communicating with the fracture, or of damage to a major blood vessel or viscus, makes the case a surgical emergency, and may influence greatly the treatment of the fracture itself. Although a nerve injury does not necessarily affect the treatment of the fracture, it is important that it be discovered at the first examination, lest the surgeon be accused later of having caused it by the treatment.

Skin wound
The presence of a skin laceration does not necessarily mean that the fracture is an open (compound) one. In some cases a laceration is incidental to the fracture and does not communicate with it. With careful examination there is seldom difficulty in deciding, from the position and nature of the wound, whether or not it communicates with the bone at the site of the fracture.

State of the circulation
The part of the limb distal to the fracture must be examined for evidence of circulatory impairment. The examination should be repeated frequently in the first 48 hours after a fresh fracture that has been immobilised in plaster or that has been operated upon: severe pain within the plaster, or marked swelling of the digits, should arouse suspicion that all is not well. The following tests, taken together, will always give the required information.

Colour. A pink colour is reassuring. A blue, grey or white colour should arouse suspicion, but in itself it does not necessarily signify circulatory impairment.

Warmth. Warm digits suggest a circulatory flow, though it may be sluggish. Cold digits do not, necessarily, bode ill, especially if the limb is encased in a fresh plaster that is still damp.

Arterial pulses. The pulses, if available for palpation, are usually a reliable guide to the state of the circulation, but when the limb is encased in plaster they are not readily accessible. If necessary, the plaster should be trimmed sufficiently to allow access to the pulses. It must be noted that in compartment syndrome, in which tension from oedema within a closed fascial compartment in the forearm or leg builds up to such an extent that the viability of the contained tissues is impaired, the pulses may be present. In such cases severe and unremitting pain is an important clue to the diagnosis, and must never be ignored. A further important feature is that impending muscle ischaemia causes severe pain when the affected muscles are stretched passively, for instance by attempting to straighten the fingers or toes when the flexor muscles are ischaemic.

Capillary return. When the digital pulp or a nail bed is compressed with a finger nail an area of blanching can be seen around the point of pressure. If on release of the pressure the blood flows back briskly into the blanched area in a pink flush, the circulation is adequate. If the return is sluggish or absent, obstruction of the circulation should be suspected. This test should be interpreted with caution, because a capillary flush (albeit less brisk than normal and dusky in colour) may be observed even when the arterial circulation is occluded, if the venous return is also obstructed. Only when the returning flush is as rapid as in the sound limb, and pink, does it testify to the integrity of the circulation.

Nerve conductivity. An ischaemic nerve quickly loses its ability to transmit impulses—a fact that can be put to advantage when examining the state of the circulation. Loss of sensibility in the digits, in the absence of physical injury to the nerves, suggests ischaemia. In deciding whether sensory impairment is caused by physical trauma to a nerve or by ischaemia it should be remembered that in ischaemic lesions all the nerve trunks in the limb are likely to be affected, whereas it is unusual for all the trunks to be involved in an injury (except in brachial plexus injuries and cauda equina injuries). Total insensibility of a hand or foot, therefore, suggests ischaemia, whereas insensibility in the territory of a single nerve denotes mechanical injury. Motor tests of nerve conductivity are less reliable than tests of sensibility because the long flexors and extensors of the digits are innervated high up in the forearm and leg and may, therefore, continue to move the digits despite complete ischaemia in the distal part of the limb.

Specific tests. If doubt still exists about the integrity of the arterial circulation, despite the clinical tests already described, resort may be had to Doppler ultrasonography or arteriography.

State of the spinal cord and peripheral nerves
Simple tests of sensibility, motor function and sweating are sufficient to indicate whether or not there has been an injury to the nervous system. Bladder function must also be investigated in suspected injuries of the spinal cord or cauda equina.

State of the viscera

Visceral injuries will give characteristic symptoms and signs which must be looked for in accordance with general surgical principles. It is particularly important to investigate the state of the bladder and urethra in every fracture involving the anterior part of the pelvis.

RADIOGRAPHIC EXAMINATION

Radiographic examination must always be insisted upon when there is any suspicion of a fracture. Although in a high proportion of cases the findings will be negative, the cost is one that must be paid for the assurance that a fracture is not overlooked. Not only is the failure to diagnose a fracture a serious matter for the patient, it is also important from the medico-legal point of view.

Radiographic technique

The standard technique is to take two projections in planes at right angles to one another—usually antero-posterior and lateral. The films should always include a good length of bone above and below the site of suspected injury, including the adjacent joints.

In special situations, additional oblique or tangential projections may be required. These are helpful particularly at sites where a fracture is notoriously difficult to detect, such as the head of the radius and the scaphoid bone. With the increasing availability of computed tomography (CT), the detection and evaluation of difficult fractures has been made much easier. Images can be viewed in three planes and even in three-dimensions, making the planning of surgical treatment much easier.

Many examples could be given to illustrate the danger of relying only on a single radiograph. If the radiographic examination is inadequate, the diagnosis of fracture or dislocation may easily be missed. For instance, in a case of posterior dislocation of the shoulder the radiograph may appear virtually normal if only an antero-posterior projection is made. This is because the humeral head, though displaced backwards out of the socket, may still cast a radiographic shadow that superimposes fairly accurately upon that of the glenoid cavity (Fig. 2.1). Only in a lateral view is it evident that the humeral head has in fact lost all contact with the glenoid cavity.

When radiographs show evidence of a fracture or dislocation, the examination should not end there. The films must be further scrutinised and, if necessary, additional films must be obtained to provide answers to the following questions:

1. Is the fracture an ordinary traumatic fracture, a fatigue fracture or a pathological fracture?
2. Are the fragments displaced, and, if so, in what direction?
3. Are the fragments in satisfactory alignment?
4. Does the fracture appear to be a recent one, and if it does not appear to be recent, is there any evidence of union?
5. Is there evidence of any associated injury, for instance of the adjacent joint or of a neighbouring bone?

Fig. 2.1 The routine antero-posterior radiograph A might be thought to show the head of the humerus normally situated in the glenoid fossa. In fact it is dislocated posteriorly. (A clue is that the arm is held in medial rotation.) Compare with the reduced position shown in B. This case exemplifies the need to obtain radiographs in two planes before the possibility of displacement can be discounted.

OTHER IMAGING TECHNIQUES

In the great majority of cases of fracture and dislocation, plain radiographs are all that are required, but there are occasions when one or more of the newer imaging techniques may add information that cannot be obtained from plain radiographs alone.

Radioisotope scanning

Bone scanning after the injection of a suitable bone-seeking isotope (usually technetium-99^{m} diphosphonate) is occasionally of value, especially when the existence of a fracture is in doubt. The presence of a fracture is evidenced by an area of increased uptake in the scan. Examples of fractures in which the diagnosis may be aided by radioisotope scanning include fractures of the scaphoid bone, and fatigue or stress fractures, particularly at unusual sites.

Computed tomography

CT scanning has an increasingly important place, particularly in the investigation of fractures of the spine and pelvis. Thus, in fractures or fracture-dislocations of the spine it can show very clearly to what extent there has been encroachment upon the spinal canal (Fig. 2.2A). High-resolution scanning is capable of revealing a fracture when it is not shown by plain radiographs. The advances that have been made in computing technology in recent years now

Fig. 2.2 Computed tomographic scans of the cervical spine. A Axial; B three-dimensional reconstruction to show complete dislocation at the C4/C5 intervertebral level. Note the double image of the vertebral body in the axial view.

allow more sophisticated imaging, with the ability to reconstruct tomographs in three planes and in three-dimensions (Fig. 2.2B).

Magnetic resonance imaging

This technique is less widely available than CT, but offers improved imaging of soft tissues, including neurological structures, and plays an important role in the assessment of spinal and pelvic fractures (Fig. 2.3). The technology is expensive, but is now available in Major Trauma Centres and allows rapid assessment of the patient with multiple injuries without the need for frequent movement and repositioning. A more recent development has been the introduction of smaller scanners that allow imaging of the arm or leg, without placing the entire patient in a whole body machine.

Clinical and radiological features of fractures

Fig. 2.3 Magnetic resonance scan of the cervical spine showing a burst fracture of the C4 vertebra with compression of the spinal cord.

TESTS OF UNION

At a certain stage in the treatment of a fracture it is necessary to ascertain whether or not sound union has occurred. The decision is made from a combination of clinical and radiological evidence. In the future it may also be possible to assess union of a long bone shaft fracture by determining the resonance of the bone electronically, or by other devices specifically designed for testing stiffness, but at present these have little practical application.

Clinical tests of union

There are three clinical tests of union:

1. **absence of mobility** between the fragments
2. **absence of tenderness** on firm palpation over the site of fracture
3. **absence of pain** when angulation stress is applied at the site of fracture (Fig. 2.4).

These tests together are reliable, but they should always be confirmed by radiological studies.

Radiological criteria of union

There are two radiological features that indicate union:

1. **visible callus bridging the fracture** and blending with both fragments (Fig. 2.5A)
2. **continuity of bone trabeculae across the fracture** (Fig. 2.5B).

Of these, visible callus is generally the earlier and the more reliable sign. Trabecular continuity across the fracture is evidence of mature union, but overlapping of the radiographic shadows of the two fragments may give a false impression of trabecular continuity when in fact it does not exist.

Fig. 2.4 Testing for union after a fracture of the tibia. The clinical signs of union are: (1) absence of movement at the fracture site; (2) absence of tenderness on palpation over the bone; and (3) absence of pain at the fracture site when stress is applied.

Fig. 2.5 Radiological criteria of union. A Bridging of the fracture by callus. B Continuity of bone trabeculae across a fracture of the scaphoid bone.

Tests of resonance

This new technique is still experimental. An intact long bone such as the tibia resonates at high frequency, whereas a bone of reduced stiffness due to healing fracture resonates at a lower frequency. As union becomes firmer the frequency gradually increases. This could become a useful method of confirming union or non-union in doubtful cases, but the variability of the soft-tissue interface may interfere with the accuracy of the method.

Principles of fracture treatment | 3

This chapter is concerned with broad principles rather than with details, but the principles can be applied, with suitable modifications, to the treatment of any fracture.

INITIAL MANAGEMENT

Before definitive treatment of a fracture is undertaken, attention must be directed to first aid treatment (Advanced Trauma Life Support (ATLS) principles), to the clinical assessment of the patient with special reference to the possibility of associated injuries or complications, and to resuscitation.

First aid
The doctor who chances to be at the scene of an accident should seldom attempt more than to ensure that the airway is clear, to control any external haemorrhage, to cover any wound with a clean dressing, to provide some form of immobilisation for a fractured limb, and to make the patient comfortable while awaiting the arrival of the ambulance.

When it is necessary to move a patient with a long-bone fracture, it will be found that pain is lessened if traction is applied to the limb while it is being moved. If it is suspected that there may be a fracture of the spinal column, special care is necessary in transport, lest injury to the spinal cord or cauda equina be caused or aggravated. It is most important to avoid flexing the spine, because flexion may cause or increase vertebral displacement, jeopardising the spinal cord. In certain types of fracture, extension is also potentially dangerous to the cord. Accordingly the patient should be lifted bodily on to a firm surface, with care to avoid both flexion and extension. If a cervical collar is available, it should be applied as a protection for the neck before moving the patient, without allowing either flexion or extension of the neck during its application.

Temporary immobilisation for the long bones of the lower limb is conveniently arranged by bandaging the two limbs together so that the sound limb forms a splint for the injured one. In the upper limb, support may be provided by bandaging the arm to the chest or, in the case of the forearm, by improvising a sling.

Haemorrhage hardly ever demands a tourniquet for its control. All ordinary bleeding can be controlled adequately by firm bandaging over a pad. Only if profuse pulsatile (arterial) bleeding persists despite firm pressure over the wound, with the patient recumbent, does the need for a tourniquet arise. Pending its application, firm manual pressure over the main artery at the root of the limb may be applied to control the bleeding. If a tourniquet is applied, those attending the patient should be made aware of the fact and of the time of its application. If necessary, a note to this effect should be sent with the patient to ensure that the tourniquet is not inadvertently left in place for too long.

If morphine or a similar drug is given at the scene of the accident a note to that effect should be sent with the patient on admission to hospital.

Clinical assessment

It must be emphasised again that an immediate assessment of the whole patient is required to exclude injuries to other systems before examination of the skeletal injury. Examination of the limb should determine:

1. whether there is a wound communicating with the fracture
2. whether there is evidence of a vascular injury
3. whether there is evidence of a nerve injury
4. whether there is evidence of visceral injury.

Resuscitation

Many patients with severe or multiple fractures, or fractures associated with other visceral injuries, are shocked on arrival at hospital. Time must be spent on resuscitation and dealing with any other life-threatening injuries before definitive treatment for the fracture is begun. Haemorrhagic shock can develop rapidly when there has been a rapid loss of a large volume of blood. The main-stay of treatment is the immediate replenishment of the circulating blood volume, either with transfused blood when time permits cross-matching, or alternatively by the use of plasma expanders and blood substitutes. Electrolytes, such as isotonic saline or Rimmer's lactate solution, can be used to establish intravenous infusion but are of little value in replacing lost blood. Colloid solutions which remain within the circulation are of more value and include dextran, a high-molecular-weight polysaccharide, gelatin solution derived from animal protein, or a plasma protein fraction solution of human albumin with a small proportion of globulin. Transfusion with colloids or whole blood is usually only required in patients with blood loss greater than 1 litre.

TREATMENT OF UNCOMPLICATED CLOSED FRACTURES

The three fundamental principles of fracture treatment—reduction, immobil-isation and preservation of function—are well known, and there is still no better way of discussing the treatment of a fracture than under these three headings.

REDUCTION

This first principle must be qualified by the words 'if necessary'. In many frac-tures reduction is unnecessary, either because there is no displacement or because the displacement is immaterial to the final result (Fig. 3.1). A con-siderable experience of fractures is needed before one can say with confidence whether or not reduction is advisable in a given case. If it is judged that perfect function can be restored without undue loss of time, despite some uncorrected displacement of the fragments, there is clearly no object in striving for perfect anatomical reduction. Indeed, meddlesome intervention may sometimes be detrimental, especially if it entails open operation.

To take a simple example, there is no object in striving to replace perfectly the broken fragments of a child's clavicle, because normal function and appearance will be restored without any intervention; the same applies to most

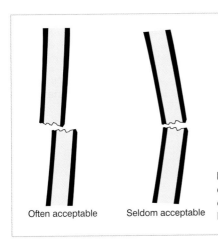

Often acceptable   Seldom acceptable

Fig. 3.1 Imperfect apposition (left) may often be accepted, whereas malalignment of more than a few degrees must usually be corrected.

fractures of the clavicle in adults. Likewise there is nothing to be gained in striving for perfect reduction of a fracture of the neck of the humerus in an elderly person—an ideal that may demand open operation for its attainment—when good or better results may be expected from conservative treatment despite imperfect reduction.

In general, it may be said that imperfect apposition of the fragments can be accepted much more readily than imperfect alignment (Fig. 3.1). For example, in the shaft of the femur a loss of contact of half a diameter might be acceptable whereas an angular deformity of 20° would usually demand an attempt at improvement. When a joint surface is involved in a fracture, the articular fragments must always be restored as nearly as possible to normal, to lessen the risk of subsequent osteoarthritis.

METHODS OF REDUCTION

When reduction is decided upon it may be carried out in three ways:

1. by closed manipulation
2. by mechanical traction with or without manipulation
3. by open operation.

Manipulative reduction
Closed manipulation is the standard initial method of reducing most common fractures. It is usually carried out under general anaesthesia, but local or regional anaesthesia is sometimes appropriate. The technique is simply to grasp the fragments through the soft tissues, to disimpact them if necessary, and then to adjust them as nearly as possible to their correct position.

Reduction by mechanical traction
When the contraction of large muscles exerts a strong displacing force, some mechanical aid may be necessary to draw the fragments out to the normal length of the bone. This particularly applies to fractures of the shaft of the femur, and to certain types of fracture or displacement of the cervical spine.

Traction may be applied either by weights or by a screw device, and the aim may be to gain full reduction rapidly at one sitting with anaesthesia, or to rely upon gradual reduction by prolonged traction without anaesthesia.

Operative reduction

When an acceptable reduction cannot be obtained, or maintained, by these conservative methods, the fragments are reduced under direct vision at open operation. Open reduction may also be required for some fractures involving articular surfaces, or when the fracture is complicated by damage to a nerve or artery. When operative reduction is resorted to, the opportunity should always be taken to fix the fragments internally to ensure that the position is maintained (see p. 43).

IMMOBILISATION

Like reduction, this second great principle of fracture treatment must be qualified by the words 'if necessary'. Whereas some fractures must be splinted rigidly, many do not require immobilisation to ensure union, and excessive immobilisation is actually harmful in some (Figs 3.2 & 3.3).

INDICATIONS FOR IMMOBILISATION

There are only three reasons for immobilising a fracture:

1. to prevent displacement or angulation of the fragments
2. to prevent movement that might interfere with union
3. to relieve pain.

Fig. 3.2 Two examples of fractures for which immobilisations is unnecessary. A Fracture of the clavicle; B undisplaced fracture of a phalanx of a finger. The fragments are held stable by the intact periosteal sheath.

Fig. 3.3 Two examples of fractures that require immobilisation. Ⓐ Fracture of the scaphoid bone; Ⓑ fracture of the neck of the femur.

If in a given fracture none of these indications applies, there is no need for immobilisation. It follows from the first of these criteria that, if reduction has been necessary, immobilisation will also be required to prevent redisplacement.

Prevention of displacement or angulation

As a general rule, the broken fragments will not become displaced more severely than they were at the time of the original injury. Therefore, if the original position is acceptable, immobilisation to prevent further displacement is often unnecessary. In fractures of the shafts of the major long bones, however, immobilisation is usually necessary in order to maintain correct alignment.

Prevention of movement

As has been mentioned already, absolute immobility is not always essential to union of a fracture. It is only when movement might shear the delicate capillaries bridging the fracture that it is undesirable, and, theoretically, rotation movements are worst in this respect. There are three fractures that constantly demand immobilisation to ensure their union—namely, those of the scaphoid bone, of the shaft of the ulna, and of the neck of the femur.

Examples of fractures that heal well without immobilisation are those of the ribs, clavicle and scapula, and stable fractures of the pelvic ring. Immobilisation is also unnecessary for certain fractures of the humerus and femur, and many fractures of the metacarpals, metatarsals and phalanges. In some fractures, excessive immobilisation may do more harm than good. The injured hand, in particular, tolerates prolonged immobilisation badly. Whereas the wrist may be immobilised for many weeks or even months with impunity, to immobilise injured fingers for a long time is to court disaster in the form of permanent joint stiffness.

Principles of fracture treatment

Relief of pain

Probably in about half of all the cases in which a fracture is immobilised the main reason for immobilisation is to relieve pain. With the limb thus made comfortable, it can be used much more effectively than would otherwise be possible.

METHODS OF IMMOBILISATION

When immobilisation is deemed necessary there are four methods by which it may be effected:

1. by a plaster of Paris cast or other external splint
2. by continuous traction
3. by external fixation
4. by internal fixation.

Immobilisation by plaster, splint or brace

For most fractures the standard method of immobilisation is by a plaster of Paris cast. Also available are various proprietary substitutes for plaster, which offer the advantages of lighter weight, radiolucency and imperviousness to water, though at much greater cost. Most such products are also more difficult to apply; nevertheless, they are being used on an increasing scale. For some fractures a splint made from metal, wood or plastic is more appropriate—for example, the Thomas's splint for fractures of the shaft of the femur, or a plastic collar for certain injuries of the cervical spine.

Plaster technique. Plaster of Paris is hemihydrated calcium sulphate. It reacts with water to form hydrated calcium sulphate. The reaction is exothermic, a fact that is evidenced by noticeable warming of the plaster during setting.

Plaster bandages may be prepared by impregnating rolls of book muslin with the dry powdered plaster, but except in a few developing countries, most hospitals now use ready-made proprietary bandages. These are best used with cold water because setting is too rapid with warm water.

Most surgeons use a thin lining of stockinet or cellulose bandage to prevent the plaster from sticking to the hairs and skin (Fig. 3.4). The use of a lining is certainly recommended because it adds greatly to the comfort of the plaster. If marked swelling is expected, as after an operation upon the limb, a more bulky padding of surgical cotton wool should be used.

The plaster bandages are applied in two forms: round-and-round bandages and longitudinal strips or 'slabs' to reinforce a particular area. Round-and-round bandages must be applied smoothly without tension, the material being drawn out to its full width at each turn. Slabs are prepared by unrolling a bandage to and fro upon a table: an average slab consists of about 12 thicknesses. The slabs are placed at points of weakness or stress and are held in place by further turns of plaster bandage.

A plaster is best dried simply by exposure to the air: artificial heating is unnecessary. A plaster will not dry satisfactorily if it is kept covered by clothing or bed-linen.

Synthetic (plastic) splinting materials are applied in much the same way as plaster bandages, usually with warm water. Since they are stronger weight for weight than plaster, fewer layers are required. Moulding to the body contours is more difficult than with plaster bandages.

Fig. 3.4 A layer of stockinet forms a comfortable lining which prevents the plaster from sticking to the hairs. An alternative is to use a single thickness of cellulose bandage. The hand is shown in a position of function, with slight dorsiflexion at the wrist and the thumb opposed.

Fig. 3.5 Technique of soaking a plaster bandage. A The end is unwound for a few centimetres so that it will be found easily when the bandage is wet. B The wet bandage is squeezed lightly from the ends but is not wrung out.

Removing a plaster. Despite the development of electrically powered oscillating plaster saws, the traditional plaster-cutting shears must still be relied upon for most plaster-cutting jobs, and it is important that correct use of the shears be fully understood. The shears act on the principle of a punch, not of scissors. There are three essential points to remember in the operation of plaster shears:

1. The line of cut should be over soft tissues and concavities and should avoid the bony prominences (Fig. 3.6).

2. The point of the shears should be slid along in the plane immediately deep to the plaster—in the case of a cotton-lined plaster, between the plaster and the lining.

3. Only one handle of the shears should be oscillated—namely the handle that is farther away from the plaster. If this rule is observed it will be found that

Fig. 3.6 Correct lines of cut for removal of plasters with the hand shears. In the forearm plaster Ⓐ the cut should be made in the midline of the anterior surface, crossing the wrist in the hollow between the tuberosity of the scaphoid bone and the pisiform bone. Only one cut is required, because the plaster is thin enough to be opened out without difficulty when it has been cut through. In the leg plaster Ⓑ two cuts should be made. The first cut should be made along the lateral surface and should pass behind the lateral malleolus, in the hollow between the malleolus and the heel. Hence it should extend along the lateral border of the sole of the foot. The second cut should be made along a corresponding line at the medial side of the plaster, passing behind the medial malleolus.

the point of the blade will be directed constantly away from the skin towards the inside of the plaster, and will remain automatically in the correct plane (Fig. 3.7).

The powered oscillating plaster saw is useful for removing a very thick plaster or synthetic cast and for cutting a window through a plaster. Oscillation rather than rotation of the blade guards against its damaging the skin, but care is needed particularly in areas where the skin is adherent to the underlying bone and not freely mobile. It is best to cut down through the plaster in multiple sections each equal to the diameter of the blade, rather than to slide the oscillating blade along the plaster (Fig. 3.8).

Fig. 3.7 The technique of operating the plaster shears. Only the handle away from the plaster (in this case the one in the surgeon's right hand) is oscillated: the other handle is held steady, parallel to the surface of the plaster. In this way the point of the blade is always directed outwards against the inside of the plaster, away from the patient's skin.

Fig. 3.8 The technique of using an oscillating saw to cut through a plaster cast.

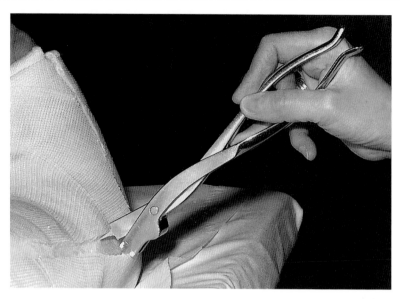

Fig. 3.9 The method of using a plaster spreader to open up the cast after it has been cut with a saw or shears.

Disadvantages of the powered saw are that it is noisy and rather frightening for the patient, and that it creates an unpleasant amount of dust.

The plaster spreader is a useful instrument with which to open up a plaster cast that has been split down one side (Fig. 3.9).

Other external splints. Apart from plaster of Paris, splints that are in general use are mostly those for the thigh and leg (Figs 3.10 & 3.11) and for the fingers. Individual splints may also be made from malleable strips of aluminium, from wire, or from heat-mouldable plastic materials such as polyethylene foam (Fig. 3.12). Rarely, a halo-thoracic splint is used for an unstable fracture of the

Fig. 3.10 Thomas's splint with Pearson knee flexion attachment, used mainly for fractures of the shaft of the femur. Note the canvas strips slung between the two bars to support the limb.

Fig. 3.11 Continuous skeletal traction through a tibial pin with balanced suspension, using a Thomas's splint and a Pearson knee flexion attachment.

Fig. 3.12 Cervical collar constructed from polyethylene foam. For more rigid support of the neck a 'halo-thoracic' splint may be used (see text).

cervical spine. This consists of a metal 'halo' or ring that is screwed to the skull and joined by bars to a plaster or plastic splint enclosing the chest (see Fig. 8.10).

Precautions in the use of plaster and splints. When a plaster has been applied over a fresh fracture, or after operation upon a limb, careful watch must always be kept for possible impairment of the circulation. Undue swelling within a closely fitting plaster or splint may be sufficient to impede the arterial flow to the distal part of the limb. The period of greatest danger is between 12 and 36 hours after the injury or operation. Severe pain within the plaster and marked swelling of the digits are warning signs that should call for a careful reassessment of the state of the peripheral circulation. The clinical tests to be applied were described on page 21.

It should be noted that after operations upon the limbs a coagulated blood-soaked dressing may act in exactly the same way as a tight plaster and may seriously obstruct the circulation.

Fig. 3.13 Ⓐ & Ⓑ Functional brace (cast brace) suitable for certain fractures of the femoral shaft or tibia. Note the plastic hinges incorporated at the knee. Hinges may also be fitted at the ankle.

If a plaster has to be split for threatened circulatory arrest it is important that it be split *throughout its length*. Dressings and bandage under the plaster should also be divided right down to the skin, and the plaster should be opened up thoroughly from top to bottom. Nothing less than this can be regarded as adequate; the consequences of half-hearted measures may be catastrophic.

Cast bracing (functional bracing). A brace has come to be understood as a supportive device that allows continued function of the part. Cast bracing, or functional fracture bracing (to use a better term), is a technique in which a fractured long bone is supported externally by plaster of Paris or by a mouldable plastic material in such a way that function of the adjacent joints is preserved and use of the limb for its normal purposes can be resumed. The technique entails snug fitting of the plaster or plastic material over the appropriate limb segments and the incorporation of metal or plastic hinges at the level of the adjacent joint (Fig. 3.13).

Functional bracing is used mainly for fractures of the shaft of the femur or tibia. Since the support that a brace gives to the fractured bone is usually less than that provided by a conventional plaster, it is prudent to defer the application of a functional brace until the fracture is already becoming 'sticky'—

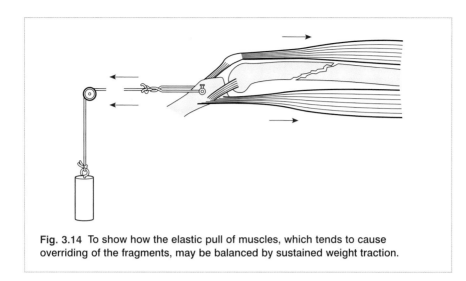

Fig. 3.14 To show how the elastic pull of muscles, which tends to cause overriding of the fragments, may be balanced by sustained weight traction.

often about 5 or 6 weeks after the injury. Earlier application of the brace may result in a recurrence of the deformity. In the meantime, treatment should be continued by sustained traction or by a conventional plaster, depending upon the nature of the fracture.

Immobilisation by sustained traction

In some fractures—notably those of the shaft of the femur and certain fractures of the shaft of the tibia or of the distal shaft of the humerus—it may be difficult or impossible to hold the fragments in proper position by a plaster or external splint alone. This is particularly so when the plane of the fracture is oblique or spiral, because the elastic pull of the muscles then tends to draw the distal fragment proximally so that it overlaps the proximal fragment. In such a case the pull of the muscles must be balanced by sustained traction upon the distal fragment, either by a weight or by some other mechanical device (Fig. 3.14). Sustained traction of this type is usually combined with some form of splintage to give support to the limb against angular deformity—usually a Thomas's splint or modified version of it in the case of a femoral shaft fracture, or a Braun's splint in the case of the tibia. The 'gallows' or Bryant method of traction for femoral shaft fractures in young children employs the principle of immobilisation by traction without any additional splintage (Fig. 15.8, p. 246). Also in this category is traction upon the skull for cervical spine injuries.

Immobilisation by external fixation

Strictly, immobilisation in plaster or in a splint might be regarded as external fixation. By convention, however, the term external fixation is used to imply anchorage of the bone fragments to an external device such as a metal bar through the medium of pins inserted into the proximal and distal fragments of a long bone fracture. In its simplest form, external fixation may be provided by transfixing each fragment with a Steinmann pin and incorporating the protruding ends of the pins in a plaster of Paris splint.

This simple method is now seldom used, and fixation is now by means of rigid bars or a frame—the fixator—to which the pins are attached by clamps with multiaxial joints. Such systems allow adjustment of the position of the fragments and, if necessary, compression of the fractured bone ends together, after the fixator has been applied. Surgeons now prefer to grip the fragments not by transfixing them through and through, but by inserting threaded pins into the bone from one side only. Two or three pins are inserted into each fragment and the protruding ends of the pins are clamped to the rigid body of the fixator, which lies just clear of the skin surface parallel with the fractured bone (Fig. 3.15A). External fixation finds its main application in the management of open or infected fractures, where the use of internal fixation devices such as plates or nails (see below) is undesirable because of the risk that it carries of promoting or exacerbating infection. The method has also gained some support as an alternative to internal fixation in the management of certain closed fractures of the long bones, particularly in the metaphyseal region.

A more specialised configuration of external fixation is the circular or Ilizarov frame (Fig. 3.15B), first pioneered in Russia but now used on a worldwide basis. It employs thinner transfixion wires, rather than pins, to secure the proximal and distal fracture fragments to the rings of the device under tension. The fixator rings are connected by more rigid threaded longitudinal rods, which can be adjusted for length and angulation. This also permits secondary procedures for the gradual correction of deformity, or even the transport of bone fragments to fill defects and restore length.

Fig. 3.15 Diagram showing the principle of two types of external fixation.
Ⓐ Unilateral frame using threaded half-pins anchored to the external bar by clamps. Ⓑ Circular (Ilizarov) frame with thinner transfixion wires attached to rings linked by adjustable rods.

Principles of fracture treatment

Immobilisation by internal fixation

Operative or internal fixation may be advised in the following circumstances:

1. to provide early control of limb fractures when conservative methods would interfere with the management of other severe injuries, for instance of the head, thorax or abdomen
2. as a method of choice in certain fractures, to secure immobilisation of the fracture and to allow early mobility of the patient, e.g. in the elderly patient with trochanteric hip fracture
3. when it has been necessary to operate upon a fracture to secure adequate reduction
4. if it is impossible in a closed fracture to maintain an acceptable position by splintage alone.

Methods of internal fixation. The following methods are currently in general use (Fig. 3.16):

1. metal plate held by screws or locking plate (with screws fixed to the plate by threaded holes)
2. intramedullary nail, with or without cross-screw fixation for locking
3. dynamic compression screw-plate
4. condylar screw-plate
5. tension band wiring
6. transfixion screws.

The choice of method depends upon the site and pattern of the fracture.

Plate and screws. This method is applicable to long bones. Usually a single six-hole plate suffices, but an eight-hole plate may be preferred for larger bones.

Fixation by ordinary plates has the disadvantage that the bone fragments are not forcibly pressed into close contact; indeed, if there is any absorption of

Fig. 3.16 Six methods of internal fixation for fractures. A Plate and screws. B Intramedullary nail (without and with locking screws). C Sliding screw-plate and screws. D Condylar screw-plate. E Tension band wiring. F Transfixion screws or Kirschner wires (for small fragments).

the fracture surfaces the plate tends to hold the fragments apart, and this may sometimes be a factor in the causation of delayed union. In order to counter this disadvantage of simple plates and to improve coaptation at the time of plating, special compression plates are available by which the fragments are forced together before the plate is finally screwed home (compression plating).

Locking plate. A newer concept is the 'locking plate', that uses screws with heads that are threaded and when tightened lock into matching threads in the holes of the plate. This produces a more rigid fixation in terms of length and angle, which is particularly valuable in comminuted fractures in osteoporotic bone. It can also be inserted with less stripping of soft tissue that preserves bone vascularity, particularly in the metaphyseal region.

Intramedullary nail. This technique is excellent for many fractures of the long bones, especially when the fracture is near the middle of the shaft. It is used regularly for fractures of the femur and tibia, and less commonly in the humerus. The original Kuntscher-type nail designed for the femur was hollow and of clover-leaf section and achieved fixation by its tight fit in the narrowest isthmus of the shaft. This type has been replaced by the newer more versatile locking nail with a rounder cross-section (Fig. 3.16), which offers notable advantages. These have transverse holes at both ends, allowing the insertion of transfixion ('locking') screws through bone and nail under image intensifier radiographic control. This affords greater rigidity as well as resistance to rotation forces allowing their use in comminuted fractures, particularly in the wider medullary canal near the bone ends. A new design of thinner more flexible solid nail is sometimes used for the management of shaft fractures in children.

Compression screw-plate. The compression screw-plate (dynamic hip screw) is a standard method of fixation for fractures of the neck of the femur and for trochanteric fractures (see Fig. 15.3). The screw component, which grips the femoral head, slides telescopically in the barrel to allow the bone fragments to be compressed together across the fracture. This compression effect is brought about by tightening a screw in the base of the barrel.

Transfixion screws. The use of a transfixion screw has wide application in the fixation of small detached fragments—for instance the capitulum of the humerus, the olecranon process of the ulna or the medial malleolus of the tibia.

Kirschner wire fixation. These thin flexible wires with sharpened ends are available in a number of diameters and provide a useful alternative to transfixion screws for the fixation of small bony fragments or for fractures of the small bones in the hand and foot.

Tension band wiring. This technique of fixation is most commonly used in the patella and olecranon, but can be applied to other small metaphyseal fragments such as the medial malleolus. It uses the mechanical principle of converting the tensile stresses of the muscles acting on the bone fragment, into a compressive force at the fracture site. This is achieved by means of tightening an eccentric figure-of-eight cerclage wire across the two fragments, stabilised by Kirschner wires or a screw inserted at right angles to the fracture line (Fig. 3.16).

Metals for internal fixation

Metals used for internal fixation of fractures or for internal prostheses must be resistant to corrosion in the tissues: silver, iron, ordinary steel and nickel-plated steel are all unsuitable. A special stainless steel containing chromium, nickel and molybdenum is widely used, but a non-ferrous alloy containing chromium, cobalt and molybdenum has even better resistance to corrosion in the body and is used for all types of internal appliance except wire, for which it is technically unsuitable. The metallic element titanium and its alloys have also proved resistant to corrosion in the body and are used increasingly for the manufacture of prostheses and internal fixation devices.

The place of operative fixation

In recent years there has been an increasing use of internal fixation for the treatment of limb fractures in most trauma centres, often as a deliberate first choice. As will be seen in a later chapter, operative fixation is already accepted as the best routine method of treating fractures of the neck and trochanteric region of the femur in the elderly. Until recently, many fractures of the shafts of the long bones have been treated conservatively—generally with excellent results, although often at the cost of rather a long time in hospital or away from work. The introduction of more sophisticated implants, inserted through small incisions under radiological screening, and offering immediate fracture fixation, has led to a dramatic change in this policy. In particular, intramedullary nailing is now used for most fractures of the shaft of the femur or tibia.

The reasons for advocating surgical intervention for fractures that were formerly managed conservatively are threefold. Firstly, there may be a substantial reduction in the time that the patient must spend in hospital and away from work. Secondly, in a favourable case function of the limb—and particularly of the joints—may be restored earlier because the need for plaster or other external splintage can often be eliminated. And thirdly, it is hoped that by providing rigid fixation of the fracture, complications such as delayed union and non-union will be reduced. In themselves, these objectives are unexceptionable, but there are arguments on the other side. The chief of these is that operative fixation, especially when combined with open reduction, entails risks that are absent or minimal with conservative treatment. Occasional fatalities—for instance from pulmonary embolism—are probably unavoidable, and major wound infection is by no means uncommon after lengthy open operations for reduction and internal fixation. Extensive stripping of soft tissues from the bone may also lead to adhesions that restrict joint movement, and may jeopardise the blood supply to the bone fragments, thereby hindering union. Thus the objects of the operation may sometimes be defeated.

It is important to strike a fair balance between these conflicting arguments, and to weigh up all the factors in every case: the age of the patient, the site and nature of the fracture, problems of employment, and economic circumstances. Advanced age should always weigh heavily in favour of an operation that will enable the patient to get out of bed sooner, whereas anything that might favour infection, such as an open wound or a pressure blister, should weigh heavily against open operation. In such cases external fixation (p. 41) as distinct from internal fixation has an important place.

The final decision on whether to use internal fixation or an alternative conservative method of fracture treatment must be made by the surgeon. They must be guided by their experience with the technique, the availability of the implants, the operating and ward environments, and the incidence of wound infection in other patients.

REHABILITATION

Improved results in the treatment of fractures owe much to rehabilitation, perhaps the most important of the three great principles of fracture treatment. Reduction is often unnecessary; immobilisation is often unnecessary; rehabilitation is always essential. In Britain, much of the credit for early enlightenment on the principles of rehabilitation must go to Watson-Jones.

Rehabilitation should begin as soon as the fracture comes under definitive treatment. Its purpose is twofold: first, to preserve function so far as possible while the fracture is uniting and second, to restore function to normal when the fracture is united. This purpose is achieved not so much by any passive treatment as by encouraging patients to help themselves.

The two essential methods of rehabilitation are active use and active exercises. Except in cases of minor injury, the patient should, ideally, be under the supervision of a physiotherapist throughout the whole duration of treatment.

Active use

This implies that the patient must continue to use the injured part as naturally as possible within the limitations imposed by necessary treatment (Fig. 3.17). The degree of function that can be retained depends upon the nature of the fracture, the risk of redisplacement of the fragments, and the extent of any necessary splintage. Although in some injuries rest may be necessary in the early days or weeks, there should be a graduated return to activity as soon as it can be allowed without risk.

Active exercises

These comprise exercises for the muscles and joints. They should be encouraged from an early stage. While a limb is immobilised in a plaster or splint, exercises must be directed mainly to the preservation of muscle function by static contractions. The ability to contract a muscle without moving a joint is soon acquired under proper supervision.

When restrictive splints are no longer required, exercises should be directed to mobilising the joints and building up the power of the muscles. Finally, when the fracture is soundly united, treatment may be intensified, movements

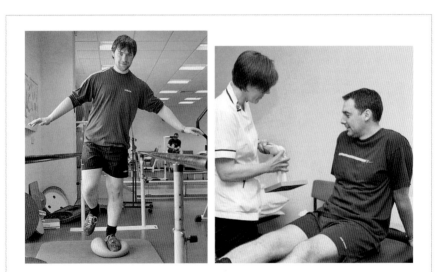

Fig. 3.17 Rehabilitation. Muscle and proprioceptive training and education.

being carried out against gradually increased resistance until normal power is regained.

Although every adult patient with a major fracture should attend for supervised exercises as often as possible, it should be impressed upon the patient that this organised treatment plays only a part in the rehabilitation, and that much—indeed most—depends upon continuing normal activities so far as possible when the patient is away from the department. Physiotherapy is often enormously helpful, but it should supplement, not supplant, the patient's own independent efforts (Figs 3.18 & 3.19).

Fig. 3.18 Rehabilitation. Class exercises for wrist and fingers.

Fig. 3.19 Rehabilitation. Exercises for active strengthening of leg muscles.

Principles of fracture treatment

So far as children are concerned, supervised exercises are relatively unimportant, and in most cases children may safely be left to their own endeavours, aided when necessary by encouragement from the parents, who should always be fully informed of the programme of treatment and the likely course of events.

Continuous passive motion

In the knowledge that movement between joint surfaces favours the preservation of healthy articular cartilage, surgeons and biomechanical engineers have designed machines that provide continuous to-and-fro movement at a joint without any effort on the part of the patient. The range of movement can be varied as required, being increased gradually as the joint becomes more mobile. This technique of exercising joints passively has many applications: it is particularly valuable in situations where restriction of mobility tends to be hard to overcome, for instance in the knee after fracture of the femoral shaft or after the operation of quadricepsplasty.

Comment

Neglect of proper rehabilitation may have serious consequences. An injured limb that is kept immobile and disused for a long period tends to suffer oedema, wasting of the muscles and stiffness of the joints, with prolonged or even permanent impairment of function. Such disasters, formerly common, are now rare where the benefits of active functional treatment are fully appreciated.

TREATMENT OF OPEN FRACTURES

An open (compound) fracture always demands urgent attention in a properly equipped operation theatre. The sooner the wound can be dealt with adequately the smaller is the risk of infection arising from contaminating organisms.

Principles of treatment

The object is to clean the wound and, whenever necessary, to remove all dead and devitalised tissue and all extraneous material, leaving healthy well-vascularised tissues that are able to ward off infection from the organisms that must inevitably remain even after the most meticulous cleansing.

The extent of the operation required depends upon the size and nature of the wound. It is important that the wound should not be subjected to repeated examination, but should be kept covered with a sterile dressing until it can be visualised under optimum conditions in the operating room. The simplest type of case is that in which there is merely a small puncture wound caused by a sharp spike of bone forcing its way through the skin. In such a case it is often clear, when the wound is carefully inspected, that there is no serious contamination, and it may be unnecessary to do more than to clean the area with water or a mild detergent solution. At the other extreme is the grossly contaminated wound of a gunshot injury, with severe tearing and bruising of the soft tissues over a wide area, and often with much comminution of the bone. Then the only hope of preventing serious infection lies in a most painstaking cleansing of the wound with the removal of all devitalised tissue, and in the avoidance of immediate skin closure.

Technique of operation for major wounds

The operation is begun by enlarging the skin wound, if this is necessary, to display clearly the extent of the underlying damage. The whole wound is then flushed with copious quantities of water or saline to remove as completely as possible all contaminating dirt: at the same time any pieces of foreign matter such as shreds of clothing are picked out with forceps. In general, the emphasis should be on thorough cleaning of the tissues rather than on drastic excision; nevertheless, tissue that is obviously dead should be excised (Fig. 3.20), and it is particularly important that dead or devascularised muscle be removed in order to reduce the risk of infection by gas-forming organisms (gas gangrene). Bone fragments that are small and completely detached may be removed, but large fragments, which usually retain some soft-tissue attachments, should be preserved. Damage to a major blood vessel is dealt with, according to circumstances, by ligation, suture or vein grafting. The ends of severed nerve trunks may be tacked lightly together with one or two sutures, to facilitate later definitive repair.

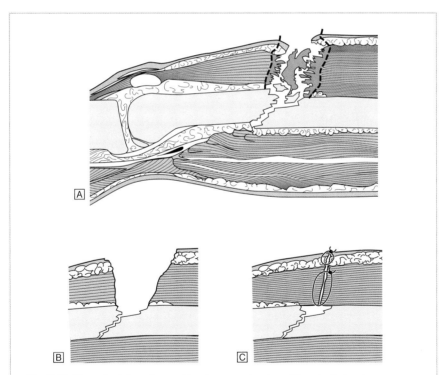

Fig. 3.20 The principles of operation for open fracture. The aim is to clean away all dirt and foreign matter and to remove dead and devitalised muscle and small loose fragments of bone, leaving the wound surfaces clean and viable. [A] Margin of necrotic tissue to be removed is shown. [B] After excision, cleansing and removal of loose bone fragments. In most cases, and invariably when there is contamination, the wound is left open until the risk of infection has subsided. It may then be closed by delayed primary suture, as in [C], or by skin grafting.

The question of skin closure

Only if a wound is of a cleanly incised type, very recent, and without any sign of contamination, may immediate suture be considered. In general, the rule should be that a major wound communicating with a fracture, in which it must be assumed that pathogenic organisms have gained entry, should never be sutured primarily. To suture such a wound, especially a gunshot wound, is to risk disastrous infection. Instead, the wound after cleansing should be left open and dressed with a sterile covering. In such a case, delayed closure may be undertaken as soon as it is clear that infection has been aborted or overcome. This technique of delayed primary suture has become standard practice in the management of high-energy gunshot wounds, which are always heavily contaminated, and the temptation to suture such a wound immediately should always be resisted.

Methods of skin closure. Whether skin closure is undertaken primarily or after an interval, the ideal method is by direct suture of the skin edges; but this is not always feasible. Whether it is practicable or not depends upon the amount of skin destroyed and lost in the injury. If the skin loss is negligible and the skin edges can be brought together without tension, direct suture should be carried out. But if the skin edges will not come together easily, the wound should be closed initially by a free split-skin graft. Where there has been extensive damage or loss of the underlying soft tissue and muscle it may be necessary to cover the bone by mobilising a muscle pedicle. Exceptionally a vascularised full-thickness graft may be required, but this more complex procedure would normally require the assistance of a specialised plastic surgical unit.

Treatment of the fracture

Once the wound has been dealt with, the treatment of the fracture itself should follow the general principles already suggested for closed fractures. The only difference is that in open fractures there should be a greater reluctance to resort to operative methods of fixation, especially if there seems to be a serious risk of infection; if it is decided that metallic internal fixation must be employed the metal should be placed well away from the wound. If the fracture is unstable and unsuitable for treatment by traction or by simple splintage alone, external fixation by pins inserted into the bone fragments and fixed to a rigid external bar (Fig. 3.15, p. 42) is often the method of choice rather than internal fixation.

Supplementary treatment in cases of open fracture

Antibiotics. A course of treatment with a broad-spectrum antibiotic, such as a third-generation cephalosporin, should be begun immediately and continued until the danger of infection is past.

Prophylaxis against tetanus. A patient who has previously been immunised against tetanus by tetanus toxoid should be given a booster dose of toxoid. If the patient has not previously been immunised it is wise to begin immunisation with a standard dose of toxoid and to follow this up with a second dose 6 weeks later.

Precautions

In severe open fractures, with perhaps considerable loss of blood, there is a greater liability to shock than there is in closed fractures, and appropriate measures of resuscitation are often required.

As with any major fracture, especially when the limb is encased in a plaster splint, careful watch must always be kept on the state of the arterial circulation, so that immediate action may be taken if signs of ischaemia should develop.

Patients treated for open fractures must be watched closely for signs that may indicate infection. The temperature chart should always be noted: any large sustained rise of temperature should be taken as an indication to inspect the wound. When there has been much contusion of muscle the possible development of gas gangrene must always be borne in mind.

Principles of fracture treatment

4 | Complications of fractures

In the great majority of fractures, union proceeds according to expectation, function of the injured part is gradually restored and little, if any, permanent disability remains. Not quite every fracture has this happy outcome. Complications inevitably occur in a proportion of them—some slight, some severe, a few catastrophic. These complications may be considered in two groups: (1) those that are concerned with the fracture itself; and (2) those that are attributable to associated injury involving other tissues. They are listed in Table 4.1.

INFECTION

Infection is virtually confined to open (compound) fractures, in which the wound is contaminated by organisms carried in from outside the body. Occasionally, a closed (simple) fracture may become infected when it is converted into an open fracture by operative intervention.

Wound infection occasionally remains superficial and the bone escapes, but more often the infection extends to the bone, giving rise to osteomyelitis. This is a serious complication because once a bone is infected with pyogenic organisms the infection tends to become chronic (Fig. 4.1A). Part of the bone may die through impairment of its blood supply, forming a sequestrum which may lie loose within a cavity in the bone for an indefinite period unless it is removed surgically. In such a case there is nearly always a persistent discharge of pus from a sinus. Infection is a potent factor in delaying or preventing union (Fig. 4.1B).

Prevention
Every effort must be made to prevent infection in cases of open (compound) fracture by prompt and meticulous cleansing and excision of all dead and

Table 4.1 Twelve complications of fractures classified into intrinsic and extrinsic groups

Complications related to the fracture itself	Complications attributable to associated injury
Infection	Injury to major blood vessels
Delayed union	Injury to nerves
Non-union	Injury to viscera
Avascular necrosis	Injury to tendons
Mal-union	Injuries and post-traumatic affections of joints
Shortening	Fat embolism
	Compartment syndrome

Fig. 4.1 [A] Osteomyelitis with purulent discharge persisting 2 years after a fracture of the tibia. [B] The radiograph shows that the fracture is still ununited. The fibula is hypertrophied because it has been supporting most of the body weight.

contaminated tissue, in the manner already described, and by the avoidance of inappropriate primary closure of contaminated wounds.

Treatment

Acute recent infection. In cases of established infection in the acute stage, the essentials of treatment are:

* to establish free drainage
* antibacterial medication.

The wound is left open and potential pockets in which pus might collect are eliminated by appropriate incision or excision of tissue. Dressings need not be frequent. Between dressings the limb is often best immobilised in plaster of Paris, or by the application of an external fixator. In a favourable case the infection is gradually overcome: indications of its quiescence are that the discharge of pus ceases and the wound becomes lined by healthy granulations. At this stage, wound closure may be attempted either by secondary suture, if practicable, or alternatively by grafting with split skin or covering with a local flap. Antibiotics should always be prescribed: a combination of flucloxacillin and fusidic acid is often appropriate, but the choice should depend upon the sensitivity of the invading organisms. The increasing incidence of methicillin-resistant strains of staphylococci in the hospital environment may necessitate the use of vancomycin, teicoplanin or lizenazolid to treat these infections effectively.

Chronic infection. If the infection of the bone passes into a persistent stage (chronic osteomyelitis), pus continues to discharge and fragments of the bone

Complications of fractures

may die and separate as sequestra. At this stage a more radical operation is required if permanent healing is to be obtained. All sequestra must be removed, and bone that is honeycombed with small pus-containing cavities must be chiselled away. Large cavities in the bone are de-roofed and 'saucerised', and they may be finally obliterated either by filling with a pedicled muscle flap or, in the case of a superficial bone such as the tibia, by lining the saucerised cavity with a split-skin graft applied direct to the raw bone. Occasionally it may be wise to excise widely the entire block of infected bone and to use distraction osteogenesis to fill the defect, a technique where the bone is divided through a distant healthy area, allowed to heal for about 7 days, and then gradually pulled apart, creating bone at this new site. Modern microsurgical techniques have allowed the use of vascularised grafts, either of bone or as a composite pedicle graft incorporating skin and muscle. This has the advantage of bringing well-vascularised tissue into the bony defect. These are particularly useful in the upper limb. However, they should not be used in the presence of active infection.

DELAYED UNION

There is no absolute time beyond which a fracture is in a state of delayed union: the borderline is arbitrary and depends to some extent upon the bone affected. As a general rule, union is deemed to be delayed if the fracture is still freely mobile 3 or 4 months after the injury. If a state of delayed union persists for many months it eventually passes into a state of non-union. The distinction between the two states is clear: whereas in delayed union there is nothing in the condition of the bones to indicate that union will fail altogether, in non-union fracture healing never will occur without further active treatment (Fig. 4.2).

Causes
The causes of delayed union are like those of non-union, but acting in less degree (see below).

Treatment
In most cases of delayed union, treatment is expectant at first, because one hopes that the fracture will eventually unite satisfactorily without surgical intervention. Patience is usually rewarded, but if union does not appear to be progressing, surgical treatment must be considered. In most such cases some form of bone grafting operation offers the best prospect of promoting union (see p. 56). In some cases, when callus has formed on both sides of the fracture, rigid internal fixation alone, without bone grafting, may be adequate.

NON-UNION

If a fracture remains ununited for many months, distinctive radiological changes take place that indicate a likely permanent state of non-union. The bone ends at the site of fracture become dense and rounded so that in contrast the fracture line itself appears increasingly clear-cut (Figs 4.1B & 4.2B). Pathologically, the process of healing appears to have come to an end, and there is no attempt to bridge the fracture with callus. Instead, the gap between the bones is filled with fibrous tissue. In some cases a cavity may form between the bone ends, i.e. an attempt to form a false joint (pseudarthrosis).

Fig. 4.2 Radiographs illustrating the distinction between delayed union (shown in the ulnar fracture in Ⓐ and non-union Ⓑ. In delayed union there is no radiographic feature to suggest that union will not occur, whereas in non-union the fractured ends of the bone are sclerotic and rounded, and there may be signs of the attempted formation of a false joint. (Another example of non-union is shown in Fig. 13.6, page 196.)

Causes

Any of the following eight factors may favour non-union:

1. infection of the bone
2. dead bone ends in association with a gap between them, i.e. incomplete reduction
3. an unfavourable mechanical environment, e.g. excessive shearing movement between the fragments
4. interposition of soft tissue between the fragments
5. loss of the fracture haematoma in an open fracture
6. dissolution of the fracture haematoma by synovial fluid (in fractures within joints)
7. medication such as non-steroidal anti-inflammatory drugs
8. destruction of bone, as by a tumour (in pathological fractures).

Sometimes two or more of these factors may act together. Acting in slighter degree, these same factors may be responsible for delayed union.

Treatment

The treatment of non-union depends upon the site of the fracture and the degree of the disability. In some cases the condition may cause only slight disability and is best left untreated—as, for instance, in certain fractures of the scaphoid bone. More often, however, non-union of a fracture is disabling and surgical treatment is desirable. Most ununited fractures of the long bones lend themselves well to treatment by bone grafting, which is usually successful in promoting union. In certain circumstances—especially when the fracture is within or near a joint—other operations may be more appropriate, such as excision of one of the fragments or its replacement by a prosthesis. In selected cases—especially when there has been loss of bone—the transfer of living bone together with its supplying and draining vessels enhances the prospects of success (see below). Other modalities such as electromagnetic stimulation, pulsed ultrasound, and injection of growth factor such as BMP morphogenetic protein have also been used.

BONE GRAFTING FOR DELAYED UNION AND NON-UNION

Bone grafts are usually obtained from another part of the patient's body (autogenous grafts). If it is impracticable or undesirable to take bone from the patient's own body, grafts obtained from another human subject may be used (allografts; homogenous grafts). These may be stored frozen or chemically preserved until required. Grafts obtained from animals (xenografts) have been used on a limited scale in recent years. Such grafts are now prepared commercially in sterile packages after elimination of their antigenic properties by deproteinisation. They have the advantage of convenience, and the discomfort to the patient entailed in taking an autogenous graft is avoided. Nevertheless, such grafts often fail to promote union of the fracture, and consequently they are little used. Autogenous grafting is much more reliable, and is the method of choice. Moreover, the use of allograft material for bone grafting is now limited by legal restrictions governing tissue banks for transplantation procedures, which require the testing of living donors for infection with pathogenic bacteria and viruses, including human immunodeficiency virus (HIV) and hepatitis virus.

Bone transferred as a free graft from one site to another does not survive in a living state. Even in a fresh graft the bone cells die, though in the case of an autogenous graft a few cells that are near the surface may possibly survive. The purpose of the graft is mainly to serve as a scaffold or temporary bridge upon which new bone is laid down. Thus the whole of a graft is eventually replaced by new living bone. This process of replacement is dependent upon adequate revascularisation of the graft, so a graft that lies in a highly vascular bed is more likely to succeed than one that is surrounded by relatively ischaemic tissue.

A modern refinement of bone-grafting techniques for recalcitrant ununited fractures is the transfer of living vascularised bone to fill a gap between the main fragments (Fig. 4.3C). This is achieved by taking the graft from a selected site together with a sizeable artery that supplies it and the draining veins, and anastomosing the vessels to appropriate vessels in the recipient area by a microsurgical technique. Such vascularised grafts, since they are composed of living bone, may be expected to become incorporated much more rapidly than non-vascularised free grafts.

BONE GRAFT SUBSTITUTES

Some synthetic substitutes for bone grafts are now becoming available for clinical use, and more are undergoing clinical trials. The reasons for their introduction are concerns about possible viral disease transmission by

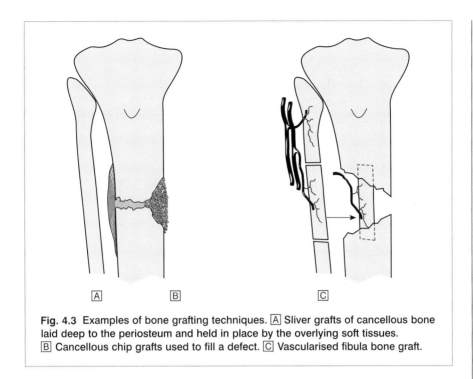

Fig. 4.3 Examples of bone grafting techniques. A Sliver grafts of cancellous bone laid deep to the periosteum and held in place by the overlying soft tissues. B Cancellous chip grafts used to fill a defect. C Vascularised fibula bone graft.

allografts, and the morbidity associated with harvesting the large quantities of autograft bone required for the treatment of major bone defects. The graft substitutes are of two types—osteoconductive and osteoinductive—but neither type combines all the biological advantages of autogenous bone. Osteo-conductive materials, such as crystalline hydroxyapatite or ceramics and calcium phosphate cements, mimic the porous structure of bone and provide a scaffold for bone cell ingrowth from the surrounding tissue. The osteoinductive materials stimulate bone healing by combining the newly isolated and genetically engineered bone morphogenetic proteins, such as BMP-2 and BMP-7, with an inert carrier of type 1 collagen. Both types of substitute have been reported to give encouraging results in the treatment of non-unions, but research continues to find the ideal synthetic material with both conductive and inductive properties.

AVASCULAR NECROSIS

Avascular necrosis (death of bone from a deficient blood supply) may have serious consequences. Not only is it sometimes a cause of intractable non-union; it also leads in many cases to disabling osteoarthritis or to total dis-organisation of a joint.

Pathology
Avascular necrosis occurs when the blood supply to a bone or part of a bone is interrupted by an injury (or, rarely, by disease). It usually occurs as a complication

Fig. 4.4 Avascular necrosis of the proximal half of scaphoid bone. A Two months after the fracture the dead fragment appears relatively dense because it has not shared in the osteoporosis from disuse that has affected the surrounding bones. B At a later stage the dead fragment is seen collapsed into an irregular mass. Osteoarthritis is inevitable.

of a fracture near the articular end of a bone, especially where the terminal fragment is devoid of vascular soft-tissue attachments and depends for its nutrition almost entirely upon the intraosseous vessels, which may be torn at the time of the injury. It may also occur after a dislocation if vital blood vessels supplying the bone are torn or occluded. In either case the immediate consequence of the ischaemia is that the bone cells die, and if the affected part of the bone lies mainly within a joint cavity (as it usually does), there is little chance that it will be revascularised from the surrounding tissues before irreversible changes of structure and form have taken place. The avascular bone gradually loses its rigid trabecular structure and becomes granular or 'gritty'. In this state the bone crumbles easily, and under the stress imposed by muscle tone or body weight it may eventually collapse into an amorphous mass (Fig. 4.4B).

This process of disintegration and collapse may sometimes be very slow: it may occur within a year of the injury or it may take as long as 3 or even 4 years. Meanwhile the overlying articular cartilage usually also dies, because its basal layers, normally nourished through vessels in the subchondral bone, are devitalised.

Thus in most cases a joint whose surface suffers avascular necrosis is doomed to crippling osteoarthritis whether or not the causative fracture eventually unites. Only in a few instances (usually in children) does the articular cartilage receive enough nourishment from the synovial fluid to enable its deeper layers to survive until the underlying bone is revascularised.

It should be noted as a point of interest that a free bone graft is necessarily avascular. Its avascularity does not create problems, however, because an articular surface is not involved. The graft becomes revascularised from the adjacent tissues and it is eventually replaced by newly formed bone.

Sites

The sites at which avascular necrosis occurs most frequently are the head of the femur after fracture of the femoral neck (p. 227) or dislocation of the hip (p. 219), the proximal half of the scaphoid bone after a fracture through the waist of the bone (p. 192), and the body of the talus after a fracture through the neck of the talus (p. 299). Sometimes an entire bone may suffer avascular necrosis after a dislocation, notably the lunate bone (p. 201).

Diagnosis

In many cases, though not in all, avascular necrosis may be recognised from radiographs about 1–3 months after the injury. Because it has no blood supply, the avascular fragment is unable to share in the general osteoporosis from disuse that affects the surrounding bones, and it stands out in sharp contrast by virtue of its relatively greater density (Fig. 4.4A).

Radioisotope scanning with technetium-99^m and magnetic resonance imaging (MRI) may also be informative if avascular necrosis is suspected. Because the affected part of the bone is devoid of blood vessels the isotope is not taken up, and consequently the avascular bone may be shown as a void area.

In the later stages, when collapse has occurred, the radiographic findings are characteristic. The bone, or the affected part of it, has lost its normal height and has a shrunken, crumbled appearance (Fig. 4.4B).

Treatment

Because of the likelihood of disorganisation of the adjacent joint, avascular necrosis often demands early operation. When collapse of the bone has not yet occurred, attempts have been made to promote revascularisation by drilling of the avascular fragment, with or without the insertion of a bone graft. In later cases it may be necessary to excise the avascular fragment and, if necessary, to reconstruct the joint by some form of arthroplasty or to stabilise it by arthrodesis.

MAL-UNION

Mal-union implies union of the fragments in an imperfect position. Thus the fragments may have united with angulation, rotation, loss of end-to-end apposition, or overlap and consequent shortening. To a slight degree, mal-union occurs in a great many fractures, but in practice the term is reserved for cases in which the resulting deformity is of clinical significance. Examples are shown in Figures 4.5 and 4.6.

It should usually be possible to prevent mal-union by competent initial treatment of the fracture, but there are occasions when some impairment of position must be accepted as inevitable despite the greatest care.

Treatment

Each case must be considered on its merits. In some cases the disability is slight and can be accepted without treatment. In others it is desirable to correct the

Fig. 4.5 Fracture of tibial shaft showing delayed union and loss of position following removal of an external fixator.

Fig. 4.6 Tibial shaft fracture with established mal-union. Note severe angulation at fracture site with loss of normal alignment between the knee and ankle joints.

deformity by dividing the bone and, after correction has been gained, fixing the fragments by the appropriate means.

SHORTENING

Shortening of a bone after fracture may arise from three causes (Fig. 4.7):

1. mal-union, the fragments being united with overlap or with marked angulation

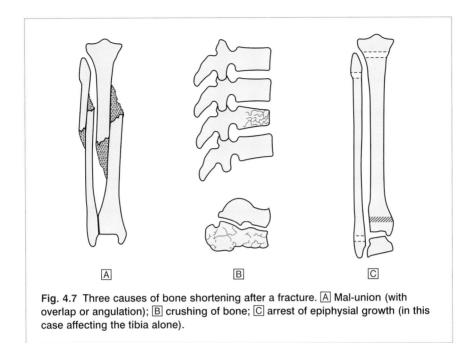

Fig. 4.7 Three causes of bone shortening after a fracture. Ⓐ Mal-union (with overlap or angulation); Ⓑ crushing of bone; Ⓒ arrest of epiphysial growth (in this case affecting the tibia alone).

2. crushing or actual loss of bone, as in severely comminuted compression fractures or in gunshot wounds when a piece of bone is shot away
3. in children, interference with the growing epiphysial cartilage (growth plate).

As a rule epiphysial growth is more likely to be impaired by a crushing injury involving the epiphysial plate than by an avulsion injury with fracture–separation of the epiphysis.

Shortening is primarily important in the lower limb. Shortening of up to 2 cm in a child is not significant and is hardly noticed. If the discrepancy is symptomatic it should be corrected by appropriate raising of the shoe, or occasionally by a leg-lengthening operation, or a leg-shortening operation on the longer side. Uncorrected shortening may cause aching in the back from tilting of the pelvis and consequent scoliosis, and also causes the patient to stand and walk with the hip on the opposite longer side adducted. This may lead eventually to discomfort in the hip, with the risk of osteoarthritis in later life.

INJURY TO MAJOR BLOOD VESSELS

Every fracture causes damage to adjacent soft tissues to some degree—especially to muscles, fascia and minor blood vessels—but in most cases the damage is repaired spontaneously along with the healing of the fracture. Occasionally an important artery is damaged, either by the agent causing the fracture (for instance, a bullet) or by the sharp edge of a bone fragment displaced at the time of the injury or subsequently. This complication may have serious consequences—indeed, it may lead to loss of the limb—but fortunately it is uncommon. The vessel may be torn across, it may be contused and occluded by thrombosis, or it may merely be temporarily sealed by spasm. The effect may be: (1) a traumatic aneurysm, or (2) impairment of blood supply in the territory of the damaged vessel with consequent gangrene, ischaemic paralysis of nerves, or ischaemic contracture of muscles (Volkmann's ischaemic contracture). It is important to remember that an equally calamitous vascular occlusion may be caused by tissue oedema within a closed fascial compartment of the forearm or leg (compartment syndrome, see p. 63), or by an overtight plaster or bandage, especially in the first 2 days after an injury or operation when swelling reaches its peak.

The most important examples of arterial injury complicating fractures and dislocations are:

- injury to the axillary artery complicating dislocation or fracture–dislocation of the shoulder
- injury to the brachial artery from supracondylar fracture of the humerus or dislocation of the elbow
- injury to the popliteal artery from dislocation of the knee or displaced fracture of the upper end of the tibia.

Rupture of the middle meningeal artery from fracture of the temporo-parietal region of the skull also comes into this category, but its management is within the province of the neurosurgeon rather than the orthopaedic surgeon.

Clinical features

The state of the peripheral circulation must be watched closely after every fracture of a long bone. The symptom that often first draws notice to ischaemia is severe pain, especially pain on attempted passive extension of toes or fingers. This must never be ignored. Numbness or loss of sensibility in the digits may also be noticed. Methods of determining the state of the peripheral circulation were described on page 21.

Treatment

A limb fracture complicated by damage to a main blood vessel must be treated urgently, because the effects of ischaemia quickly become irreversible. The treatment depends upon whether the occlusion is primary (signs of ischaemia present when the patient is first received) or secondary (ischaemia becoming apparent after reduction and immobilisation of the fracture).

If the arterial injury is evident when the patient is first received it must be assumed that the vessel has been occluded by direct injury. The following action must be taken:

- **First step.** Any external splint or bandage that might be causing constriction is removed, and gross displacement of the fragments, if not already reduced, is corrected so far as possible by gentle manipulation. If these measures fail to bring about a return of adequate circulation within half an hour the next step is taken.
- **Second step.** At operation the damaged artery is exposed and the nature of the injury determined. If the occlusion is due to kinking or spasm of the artery an attempt is made to relieve it by freeing the vessel. If this fails, the artery may be distended by the injection of heparinised saline between clamps. If the vessel is found to be divided or punctured it may be

possible to restore patency by direct suture of the freshened ends, and when there is extensive occlusion by thrombosis following damage to the intima this may be combined with endarterectomy. Alternatively, it may be practicable to excise the damaged segment and to effect repair with a vein graft. When the artery has been dealt with, the fracture should usually be fixed internally to prevent the possibility of further vascular damage from recurrent displacement.

If vascular occlusion becomes evident only after the fracture has been reduced and immobilised in plaster, no time should be lost before splitting the plaster and the underlying dressings *throughout their whole length*, and opening up the plaster thoroughly right down to the skin. If this fails to restore the circulation within half an hour the affected artery should be explored and dealt with as outlined above.

COMPARTMENT SYNDROME

Muscles are enclosed within fascial compartments, and if swelling occurs within a compartment as a consequence of an injury, a vicious circle is set up: the swelling occludes the smaller arteries or veins supplying the muscles, and the muscle ischaemia in turn promotes further swelling. Within a few hours irreversible changes may occur: the muscles may become necrotic and the nerves within the affected compartment lose their conductivity because of ischaemia. The muscles are eventually replaced by fibrous tissue, which threatens to produce a disabling contracture (Volkmann's ischaemic contracture) seen most often in the flexor muscles of the forearm or lower leg. It is important to remember that in compartment syndrome the peripheral arterial pulses may still be present and this may deflect the unwary from the true diagnosis.

Treatment
Incipient compartmental ischaemia of this type, denoted by severe pain especially on attempted passive extension of the digits, demands immediate operation to decompress the whole length of the affected compartment or compartments by fasciotomy.

INJURY TO NERVES

Peripheral nerves are injured by fractures much more often than major arteries. Well-recognised sites at which a nerve is liable to be damaged are shown in Figure 4.8.

Nerve injuries have been classified into three types: neurapraxia, axonotmesis and neurotmesis. In *neurapraxia* the damage is slight and causes only a transient physiological block. Recovery occurs spontaneously within a few weeks. In *axonotmesis* the internal architecture of the nerve is preserved, but the axons are so badly damaged that peripheral degeneration occurs. Recovery can occur spontaneously, but it depends upon regeneration of the axons and may take many months (2–3 cm per month is the usual speed of regeneration). In *neurotmesis* the structure of the nerve is destroyed by actual division or severe scarring. Recovery is possible only after excision of the damaged section, with end-to-end suture of the stumps or bridging by a nerve graft.

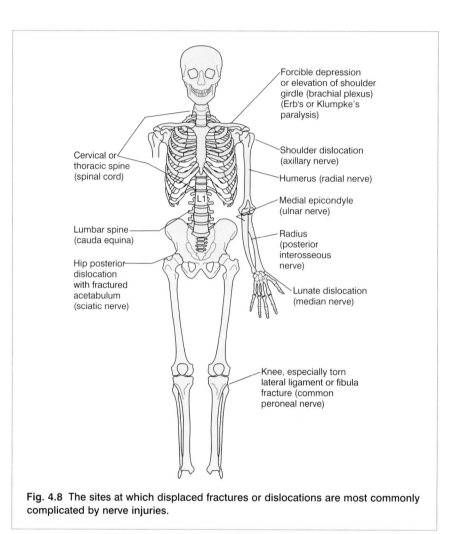

Forcible depression or elevation of shoulder girdle (brachial plexus) (Erb's or Klumpke's paralysis)

Cervical or thoracic spine (spinal cord)

Shoulder dislocation (axillary nerve)

Humerus (radial nerve)

Medial epicondyle (ulnar nerve)

L1

Lumbar spine (cauda equina)

Radius (posterior interosseous nerve)

Hip posterior dislocation with fractured acetabulum (sciatic nerve)

Lunate dislocation (median nerve)

Knee, especially torn lateral ligament or fibula fracture (common peroneal nerve)

Fig. 4.8 The sites at which displaced fractures or dislocations are most commonly complicated by nerve injuries.

In closed injuries the nerve is usually contused by the sharp edge of a bone fragment but retains its continuity. The lesion may be a neurapraxia or an axonotmesis, and spontaneous recovery is to be expected. Occasionally the nerve is severed (neurotmesis). In open fractures, especially those caused by penetrating injuries, the nerve is more often severed by the agent causing the fracture than by the bone edge itself.

Treatment

In closed injuries it may usually be assumed that the nerve is in continuity, and spontaneous recovery may be awaited with reasonable confidence. If the first signs of recovery are not observed within the expected time (calculated from the site of injury and length to be regenerated, on the assumption that a regenerating nerve fibre will grow at the rate of 2–3 cm per month) exploration is advised so that, if the nerve is found divided or badly scarred, it may be repaired.

In open fractures caused by a transfixion or piercing injury, if nerve function is lost it should be assumed that the nerve is severed. The wound should be explored and the nerve identified. If it is severed, the ends should be tacked together lightly with one or two sutures but definitive repair of the nerve should be postponed until the wound is healed, because the divided ends are seldom sufficiently cleanly cut to permit primary repair. The best time for secondary nerve repair is 3 or 4 weeks after the injury, provided the state of the wound permits. At that time the extent of the scarring, and consequently the length of nerve to be resected, can be determined accurately, and thickening of the nerve sheath makes suture technically easier. Despite these guidelines, it should be noted that when adequate facilities and skill are available, primary repair of a divided nerve may be undertaken provided the wound is clean, recent and not contaminated.

The treatment of injuries of the spinal cord and cauda equina is considered on page 122.

INJURY TO VISCERA

Like arteries and nerves, viscera may be damaged either by the agent causing the fracture or by impalement upon a sharp fragment of bone. Examples are: laceration of pleura or lung complicating fractures of the ribs; and rupture of the bladder or urethra, or penetration of the colon or rectum, complicating fractures of the pelvis. It should be noted that the spleen or a kidney, and occasionally the liver, may be ruptured by direct trauma to the trunk without fracture.

Treatment
The treatment of visceral injuries complicating fractures should follow general surgical principles; because of the risk to life that attends such injuries, their treatment must take precedence over the treatment of the fracture.

INJURY TO TENDONS

In open fractures tendons may be severed by the agent causing the fracture. Treatment is by surgical reconstruction. Delayed rupture of the tendon of extensor pollicis longus is a well-known complication of fracture of the lower end of the radius (p. 185).

INJURIES TO JOINTS

Acute joint injuries such as dislocation, subluxation or ligamentous strain are common complications of fractures. These injuries will be considered separately in Chapter 7.

INTRA-ARTICULAR AND PERI-ARTICULAR ADHESIONS

Joint stiffness from adhesions is common after fractures, especially those that are near a joint. Some joints are much more vulnerable in this respect than others. Thus the knee, shoulder, elbow and finger joints stiffen easily and often suffer permanent impairment, whereas the hip and wrist usually regain their full mobility without difficulty.

Fig. 4.9 Impaired range of knee movement 6 months after a fracture of the shaft of the femur. Stiffness is caused more often by peri-articular and intramuscular adhesions, or by adhesion of muscle to the underlying bone, than by adhesions within the joint itself.

Intra-articular adhesions occur chiefly after a fracture that has involved the articular surface of a bone. Blood escapes into the joint (haemarthrosis) and, although such an effusion can be absorbed completely without causing ill effect, it may leave residual strands of fibrin which later become organised into fibrous adhesions between opposing folds of synovial membrane.

Peri-articular changes are a more frequent cause of joint stiffness than intra-articular adhesions (Fig. 4.9). In consequence of the injury itself, and of possibly prolonged immobilisation, oedema fluid collects in the tissues, binding together the connective tissue fibres. This leads to loss of resilience of the peri-articular tissues such as joint capsule and ligaments, and in the case of muscles it impairs the free gliding of the fibres one upon another. A further common factor in the causation of stiffness is direct adhesion of muscle to the underlying bone at the site of fracture.

Joint stiffness complicating fracture should so far as possible be prevented by early mobilisation of the adjacent joints.

Treatment

Joint stiffness from the causes mentioned will nearly always respond well to active exercises, preferably carried out under the supervision of a physiotherapist. The exercises may have to be continued for a long time, often for many months, before the greatest restoration of movement is gained.

Manipulation. In the occasional case in which steady improvement is not being gained by exercise and active use, manipulation under anaesthesia may be considered. In general, manipulation is more likely to be successful in overcoming stiffness from intra-articular adhesions (that is, after direct injury or operation upon the joint) than in cases of peri-articular or muscular rigidity. Manipulation should seldom be recommended until active exercises have had a thorough trial for at least 2 months, and usually longer.

Caution. Manipulation for joint stiffness should be carried out with extreme care. A bone may easily be fractured if excessive force is used, especially in an elderly patient. The patella, in particular, is easily broken during manipulation for stiffness of the knee, and the humerus during manipulation of the shoulder. Great force should never be used: it is better to gain slight improvement by repeated gentle manipulation than to rely upon a single forcible movement.

Operation. If the joint stiffness is severe and resistant to prolonged conservative treatment then an attempt to free the joint by operation may have to be considered. For intra-articular adhesions it may be possible to carry this out arthroscopically. For extra-articular adhesions, such as those that result in intractable stiffness of the knee from adhesions of the quadriceps muscle after fracture of the distal the femur, may require open release (quadricepsplasty) (p. 248).

POST-TRAUMATIC OSSIFICATION

Post-traumatic ossification—sometimes called myositis ossificans[1]—is a rare cause of joint stiffness after a fracture or dislocation. It occurs only in cases of severe injury to a joint, and especially when the capsule and periosteum have been stripped from the bones by violent displacement of the fragments. Blood collects under the stripped soft tissues, forming a large haematoma about the joint. Instead of being absorbed, the haematoma is invaded by osteoblasts and becomes ossified (Fig. 4.10). If a large mass of bone is formed, the consequent restriction of joint movement may be severe.

This complication is encountered most commonly in the elbow after fracture–dislocation. It is also well recognised in the hip after dislocation. There is a greater risk of its occurrence in children than in adults because in children the periosteum is only loosely attached to the long bones and is easily stripped from them. There is also a relatively high incidence, often at the joints of the lower limbs, in patients with prolonged or permanent brain damage from head injury, and in patients with paraplegia from spinal injuries.

Treatment

After a severe injury of a joint, and especially of the elbow in children, the risk of the formation of a large haematoma should be minimised by enforcing complete rest for the joint, preferably in a plaster, for 3 or 4 weeks. In an established case of para-articular ossification with limitation of joint movement, treatment at first should consist only of gentle active exercises, with avoidance of strains or stretching that might provoke further bleeding beneath the soft tissues. After several months it may be justifiable to excise a mass of bone that is blocking movement, but the operation is not always successful and it must be approached with caution. In joint stiffness from this cause, manipulation is likely to do more harm than good and it should be avoided.

---

[1] The use of the term myositis ossificans to denote post-traumatic ossification about a joint should be avoided. Ossification occurs deep to the muscles and is not associated with an inflammatory lesion of the muscles, as the name implies.

Complications of fractures

Fig. 4.10 Post-traumatic ossification about the elbow after a severe fracture–dislocation. The ossification has occurred in the haematoma beneath the stripped-up periosteum and capsule.

REFLEX SYMPATHETIC DYSTROPHY
(Sudeck's[2] atrophy; Sudeck's post-traumatic osteodystrophy; post-traumatic painful osteoporosis; Complex regional pain syndrome)

Reflex sympathetic dystrophy, or post-traumatic painful osteoporosis, is an occasional cause of prolonged disability after fractures or other injuries of the limbs. It is characterised by pain, swelling and marked joint stiffness in the hand or foot of the injured limb. The cause and exact nature of the condition are unknown, but it probably results from a disturbance of centrally mediated autonomic regulation with consequent increased stimulation of sympathetic and motor efferent fibres.

Clinical features
The symptoms are noticed about 2 months after the injury, or when the plaster is removed. The function of the limb is not regained as it should be with active use and exercises. Instead, the patient complains of severe pain in the affected hand or foot when attempting to use it. On examination, the extremity is

---

[2] Paul Hermann Sudeck, a German surgeon, described a type of acute bone atrophy in 1900. In fact, however, he was referring to acute inflammatory bone atrophy rather than to post-traumatic atrophy.

Fig. 4.11 Ⓐ Sudeck's atrophy affecting the hand after a Colles's fracture. Note the patchy loss of density. A normal hand is shown in Ⓑ for comparison. The osteoporosis comes on more rapidly and is more extreme than the osteoporosis of disuse, and the bone changes are accompanied by oedema, glazing of the skin and marked stiffness of the joints.

swollen and may be hyperaemic. The skin creases are obliterated, giving the surface a glossy appearance. The nails and hair of the hand or foot are atrophic. The palmar aponeurosis may be thickened. Joint movements are severely impaired, especially the metacarpo-phalangeal and interphalangeal joints in the case of the hand ('frozen hand'). Radiographs show spotty osteoporosis, often of severe degree (Fig. 4.11).

Diagnosis
Reflex sympathetic dystrophy has features that distinguish it from the osteoporosis that is commonly seen in limbs immobilised for a long time. In particular, the marked swelling, glossy stretched appearance of the skin and marked stiffness of the joints are characteristic. In addition, the rarefaction of the bones, often with a spotty texture, is more extreme. A radioisotope bone scan may show a diffuse area of increased uptake in the affected region.

Treatment
Most cases respond slowly but surely to efficient conservative treatment. The mainstay of treatment is active exercise, with active use of the limb so far as the pain will allow. These measures may be aided by periods of elevation and local heat in the form of warm baths. Much patience and encouragement are

required, and the patient should be under the care of a skilled physiotherapist. With conservative treatment on these lines, adequate recovery is usually gained in 2–4 months.

In obstinate cases success has been claimed for intravenous infusions of guanethidine to produce regional sympathetic blockade. However, recent randomised trials have failed to show significant improvement. Failing this, resort may be had to repeated regional sympathetic block by injection of local anaesthetic solution.

OSTEOARTHRITIS
(osteoarthrosis; degenerative arthritis)

Any roughening or irregularity of a joint surface is liable to precipitate the wear-and-tear changes that form the basis of osteoarthritis. Osteoarthritis, therefore, is likely to develop sooner or later after any displaced fracture which involves an articular surface unless the fragments can be replaced so perfectly in position that the smooth contour of the joint surface is unimpaired (Figs 4.12 & 4.13). Even a slight step between the fragments may lead to serious subsequent disability from arthritis, especially in a weight-bearing joint.

Avascular necrosis as a cause of severe osteoarthritis or of total disorganisation of a joint was discussed on page 57.

Even in fractures that do not directly involve a joint surface there is a risk of later osteoarthritis if the fragments unite with angular deformity, throwing the joint out of its correct alignment, because mal-alignment of joint surfaces

Fig. 4.12 Osteoarthritis of the wrist complicating an ununited fracture of the scaphoid bone. Note the spurring of the margins of the radio-scaphoid joint, and narrowing of articular cartilage.

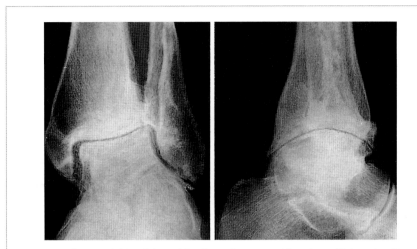

Fig. 4.13 Osteoarthritis of the ankle after a fracture-subluxation with incongruity and tilting of the joint surfaces. Note the marked narrowing of the joint space, indicating loss of articular cartilage.

causes excessive stress at one part of the joint and consequently accelerates wear-and-tear changes. An example of osteoarthritis developing in these circumstances is osteoarthritis of the knee due to bow-leg deformity after a mal-united fracture of the femoral shaft (Fig. 4.14).

As would be expected, the risk of osteoarthritis after a fracture varies according to the severity of the residual damage to the joint. The risk is much greater in the weight-bearing joints of the lower limb than in the relatively lightly stressed joints of the upper limb.

The interval between the fracture and the development of osteoarthritis also varies widely. After severe damage to a joint, osteoarthritis may become clinically evident within 6 or 9 months of the injury, whereas in cases of slight damage or mal-alignment it may not become apparent for 15 or 20 years or more.

FAT EMBOLISM SYNDROME

Fat embolism syndrome, though uncommon, is one of the most serious complications of fractures and despite recent improvements in management it is still often fatal. The essential feature is occlusion of small blood vessels by fat globules.[3]

---

[3] There is histological evidence that fat embolism occurs in minor degree very commonly after fractures: usually it does not cause symptoms. Here the term fat embolism is used only for those cases in which clinical features are evident, presumably from small vessel occlusion on a massive scale.

Fig. 4.14 [A] Old fracture of femoral shaft which united with excessive lateral bowing. (The old-time plate and screws were evidently of unsuitable metal, because they have partly disintegrated.) [B] Corresponding knee of the same patient 20 years after the fracture, showing advanced osteoarthritis. There is always a liability to osteoarthritis when the line of weight transmission through a hinge joint is shifted laterally or medially.

Pathology

Occlusion of small vessels has its most significant effects in the lungs and brain. In the lungs there are oedema and haemorrhages in the alveoli, so that transfer of oxygen from alveoli to arterioles is impaired. This leads to hypoxaemia, which may be severe. In the brain there may be multiple petechial haemorrhages. Petechial haemorrhages occur also in other organs and in the skin.

Clinical features

Fat embolism syndrome occurs mainly after severe fractures in the lower limbs, particularly those of the femur and tibia. The onset is usually within 2 days of injury, but it is notable that there is a symptom-free period between injury and onset—an important point of distinction from cerebral contusion. The presenting feature is breathlessness, usually associated with cerebral disturbance in the form of marked restlessness, confusion, drowsiness or coma. These cerebral symptoms may be caused partly by petechial haemorrhages in the brain, but in large measure they are probably secondary to hypoxia from occlusion of small vessels in the lungs. Associated features are tachypnoea and dyspnoea. The other common clinical manifestation is a petechial rash, usually on the front of the neck, anterior axillary folds or chest, or in the conjunctiva. The finding of such a rash strongly supports a diagnosis of fat embolism syndrome.

Diagnosis

Apart from the characteristic clinical features, the most important diagnostic investigation is arterial blood gas analysis. This may show reduction of the partial pressure of oxygen in the blood (PO_2) well below the normal 100 mmHg and often below the critical level of 60 mmHg at which respiratory failure is likely.

Treatment

Fat embolism is spontaneously reversible if the patient can be tided over the dangerous period of hypoxia. This may usually be corrected by the administration of 100% oxygen, if necessary with positive pressure respiration. The oxygen requirement should be controlled by repeated blood gas analysis. The administration of methylprednisolone in patients with severe multiple injuries may help to prevent and correct the adverse effects of fat embolism by maintaining blood oxygen tension and stabilising the free fatty acids. Heparin or Dextran 40 may also be administered intravenously to improve capillary flow.

5 | Special features of fractures in children

It has been mentioned already that in some respects fractures behave differently in children and in adults. The differences are mostly not fundamental but are rather differences of degree, with the exception of injuries to the growth plate.

PATHOLOGY

Injuries involving the growth plate

The most obvious difference between the bones of children and those of adults is the presence in childhood of cartilaginous growth plates at each end of the major long bones but usually at only one end of the 'short' long bones (metacarpals and metatarsals). Here it may be recalled that the greater proportion of the growth of the bone, and later closure of the growth plate, occurs in the humerus at the proximal end, in the radius and ulna at the distal end, in the femur at the distal end, and in the tibia and fibula at the proximal end. In other words, the most growth occurs 'away from the elbow and towards the knee'.

The growth plate is a potentially weak point in the bone, and at certain sites the epiphysis may be avulsed, in part or totally, from the metaphysis of the shaft. Typically, a corner of the metaphysis is carried with a displaced epiphysis (Fig. 5.1). Such an avulsion injury is usually caused by a rotational or angulatory force. In contrast, direct injury may sometimes lead to crushing of the growth plate. These epiphysial injuries and displacements are common at the proximal and distal ends of the humerus, femur and tibia, where they may result in arrest or distortion of normal growth at the plate. Their recognition and differentiation from the normal epiphysis are important and have led to a special radiological classification (Fig. 5.2).

Radiological classification

- Type I injury: complete separation of epiphysis at the growth plate without damage to the metaphysis or epiphysis.
- Type II injury: the most common type, with a characteristic triangular fragment of the metaphysis attached to the displaced epiphysis.
- Type III injury: involves the articular surface with separation of an epiphysial fragment.
- Type IV injury: fracture of the articular surface with extension across the growth plate into the metaphysis.
- Type V injury: compression fracture involving part or all of the growth plate.

Bone resilience

In childhood the long bones also differ from the adult state in that they are more resilient and springy, withstanding greater deflection without fracture.

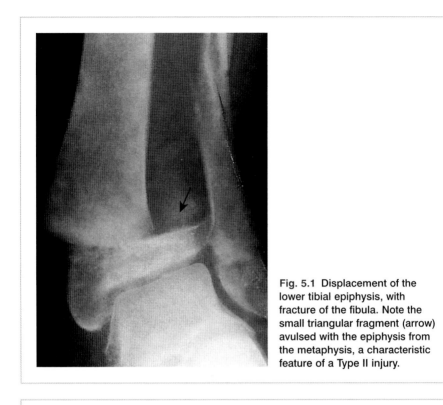

Fig. 5.1 Displacement of the lower tibial epiphysis, with fracture of the fibula. Note the small triangular fragment (arrow) avulsed with the epiphysis from the metaphysis, a characteristic feature of a Type II injury.

Fig. 5.2 Salter–Harris classification of epiphysial injuries (see text).

This accounts for the frequency—in young children, a predominance—of incomplete fractures of the greenstick type (p. 6). Such fractures do not occur in adults.

Periosteum
Another striking feature of children's bones is that the periosteum is attached only loosely to the diaphysis and, in consequence, it is easily stripped from the bone over a considerable part of its length by blood collecting beneath it. This subperiosteal haematoma is soon replaced by callus, which therefore is often seen to extend a long way up or down the shaft, even when there has been little displacement of the fragments.

Site of fracture
In the matter of sites of fracture, children present similarities to, and differences from, adults. In both children and adults, fractures of the lower forearm, clavicle, tibia and fibula are among the most common injuries. But in children, unlike adults, fractures of the scaphoid bone and neck and trochanteric region of the femur are uncommon. On the other hand, serious fractures of the elbow region (especially supracondylar fractures and fractures of the capitulum of the humerus) are relatively common, and, indeed, they present some of the most difficult problems of all childhood injuries.

Healing
Healing of childhood fractures is nearly always rapid, and the younger the child the more rapid the healing. In infancy a fracture may be soundly united in 2 or 3 weeks. In later childhood the average time required for union gradually increases, and after growth has ceased age has little effect upon the rate of union.

Remodelling
Similarly, remodelling is very active and complete in early childhood; so much so that all evidence of a past fracture may be obliterated within a matter of months (see Fig. 1.7, p. 11). It must be remembered, however, that remodelling can never fully restore a joint surface to its normal alignment if it has been tilted sideways by angulation at the site of fracture (Fig. 5.3).

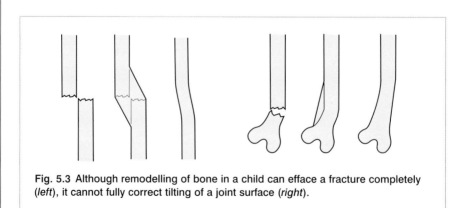

Fig. 5.3 Although remodelling of bone in a child can efface a fracture completely (*left*), it cannot fully correct tilting of a joint surface (*right*).

Effect on growth

After a fracture of a long bone in a child, growth is often accelerated for a time, perhaps from hyperaemia of the neighbouring epiphysial cartilage, but any consequent discrepancy of length is slight and of no clinical significance. On the other hand, growth may be seriously disturbed if the growth plate (epiphysial cartilage) is damaged in such a way that a bony bridge is formed across the plate between epiphysis and diaphysis, leading to premature epiphysial fusion.

If the whole area of the growth plate is fused, all growth ceases at that particular site. The degree of consequent shortening of the bone will then depend upon the age at which premature fusion occurs: the younger the patient at the time of fusion, the greater the eventual shortening.

If premature fusion occurs in only a part of the epiphysial plate, further growth will be prevented at that point but will continue in the undamaged part of the plate, thus leading to angulation deformity (Fig. 5.4A). Angulation will also occur if there is premature arrest in one bone of a pair, as in the forearm or lower leg. Thus, for instance, if growth is arrested at the lower epiphysis of the fibula but continues in the corresponding epiphysis of the tibia, the ankle region will be bowed into valgus (Fig. 5.4B).

In general, fractures that damage the growth plate in such a way as to cause premature fusion tend to be of the crushing type, whereas avulsion injuries are less likely to have that effect.

When premature bony bridging across a growth plate occurs at an early age, it is sometimes possible to prevent uneven growth by timely operative excision of the bone bridge, the gap being filled by a graft of fatty tissue.

Fig. 5.4 [A] Premature fusion at one part of the growth plate, with continuation of growth elsewhere, leads to angular deformity. [B] Bowing will also occur if epiphysial arrest occurs in only one bone of a pair.

DIAGNOSIS

Recognition of a fracture may be more difficult in a child than in an adult. As a rule, complete fractures do not present any special difficulty, but an incomplete fracture is sometimes overlooked because the more dramatic signs of fracture are often absent. Thus there may be no deformity, no abnormal mobility, no crepitus. Moreover, a history of injury is not always forthcoming, especially in young children unable to speak for themselves. Sometimes, indeed, the parents or guardians attempt deliberately to conceal the fact that an infant has been injured, especially when there has been ill-treatment ('battered baby syndrome' or 'non-accidental injury'). Recognition of the true nature of the case may then be difficult, even with the aid of radiographs, because these infantile fractures often affect the metaphysial regions of the long bones, they are often multiple, and they may produce abundant callus. The radiographic appearance may thus be atypical, and confusion may arise with such conditions as scurvy, syphilis, osteomyelitis or bone tumours. Irrespective of the history, the possibility of injury should always be considered when marked loss of function or unwillingness to use a limb is associated with local pain and tenderness.

COMPLICATIONS

Complications of fractures in children are broadly similar to those that occur in adults, though the incidence is different. Failure of union is very unusual in children, except in fractures at one particular site, namely the capitulum of the humerus. Complications in the form of avascular necrosis of the femoral head and non-union are also well recognised after fracture of the neck of the femur, though this itself is an unusual injury in children. In general, other complications are less frequent than in adults, but two that are important and relatively common require special mention: injury to the brachial artery complicating supracondylar fracture of the humerus, and post-traumatic ossification about the elbow after a displaced fracture or dislocation. This latter complication may lead to severe restriction of movement at the elbow.

An important complication that is peculiar to children is disturbance of growth after injuries involving the growth plate. The effects of such injuries have already been discussed (p. 77). Treatment is often required for the prevention or correction of deformities arising from epiphysial injuries.

Osteoporosis and fragility fractures | 6

Osteoporosis is a common disease in the elderly and is now recognised as the major contributory factor to the rising number of so-called 'fragility fractures' in this age group. As a result of this condition 40% of women and 14% of men over the age of 50 will suffer a fracture. With the increasing number of elderly people, it is anticipated that this disease process will become an epidemic in the years to come. Indeed, it has been predicted that by the year 2050 there will be 6.5 million hip fractures worldwide.

The condition is characterised by loss of trabecular bone mass and connectivity as well as thinning of cortical bone. Low bone mineral density in the elderly can result from either low peak bone mass or accelerated bone loss, or a combination of the two. A strong genetic component has also been suggested, contributing to the pathogenesis of fragility fractures. Caucasians are more vulnerable to osteoporotic fracture than other races.

Osteoporosis increases the number of fragility (low energy) fractures and contributes to the severity of traumatic (high energy) fractures. The three commonest fragility fractures are the Colles fracture of the distal radius, the femoral neck or 'hip' fracture, and crush fractures of the thoracic and lumbar vertebrae. The management of these fractures is difficult due to poor bone stock, which reduces the strength of fixation of implants used for stabilisation of the fracture. In particular, fixation of fractures affecting the metaphyseal region of long bones can be associated with an increased risk of complication such as non-union, malalignment, metalwork failures, and re-operation. After vertebral fractures, there is a major reduction in quality of life and patients suffer from back pain, depression, disability and loss of height. There is also a significant morbidity associated with fragility fractures, particularly those of the hip; these patients have an excess mortality of 20%.

PATHOGENESIS

Bone consists of an organic component (primarily cells, blood vessels and proteins such as collagen), and an inorganic mineral component, primarily a crystalline calcium phosphate compound (hydroxyapatite). In the disease of osteomalacia (termed 'rickets' in children), this mineral phase is deficient and is commonly due to insufficient calcium or Vitamin D intake. Conversely, osteoporosis is a disease in which both organic and inorganic components are deficient, resulting in a decrease in the total bone mass. As a result of this, the micro-architecture is disrupted, with loss of trabeculae and an increase in the size of the pores/spaces within the bone (Fig. 6.1 of normal, osteoporotic and osteomalacic bone).

Osteoporosis and fragility fractures

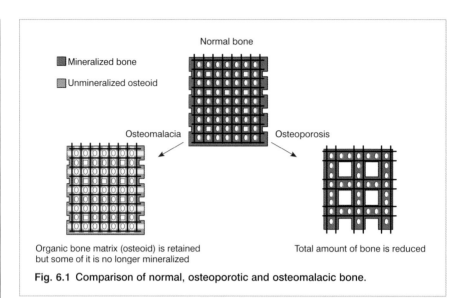

Fig. 6.1 Comparison of normal, osteoporotic and osteomalacic bone.

DEFINITION

Osteoporosis is a loss of bone mass to the level below the range of an individual of a similar race and sex. The World Health Organization has defined osteoporosis as an individual whose bone mass is more than two and a half times below that of a young adult of the same sex. Individuals with levels lower than normal, but within 2.5 standard deviation, are referred to as 'osteopenic' (Table 6.1).

Table 6.1   Causes of osteoporosis

Hereditary Osteogenesis imperfecta
Rheumatological Rheumatoid arthritis Ankylosing spondylitis
Disuse Paralysis, paraplegia, tetraplegia Polio
Respiratory Chronic obstructive lung disease
Hormonal Hypogonadism Cushing's disease (hypercortisolism)
Lifestyle Alcoholism Smoking
Drugs Steroids

MECHANISM OF FRACTURE

In the normal metaphysis the cortex is thinner than in the diaphysis. A large amount of the strength of the bone resides in the cancellous bone of the metaphysis. With osteoporosis there is a more pronounced loss of the cancellous bone than the cortical bone and therefore the bone is particularly weak in the metaphyseal region. For this reason fragility fractures commonly occur in the region of the metaphysis of long bones, or in axial bones composed largely of cancellous bone. The common sites include the hip (proximal femur), wrist (distal radius), the vertebral bodies, ankle, proximal humerus, and pelvis (pubic rami).

CHANGES IN BONE MASS WITH AGE

Bone mass increases during the growth of childhood and reaches a peak in young adult life. The level of this peak is dependent on hereditary factors (estimated to account for 70% of the variation) and environmental factors; such as the level of physical activity during childhood and adolescence, the age of the menarche, as well as the amount of calcium and milk intake. The response of the skeleton to exercise is most marked during the phase of rapid growth. It is therefore vital that children take part in exercise so that they achieve an adequate peak bone mass. The bone mass remains relatively constant during early life, but then at approximately 50 years an age-related loss of bone starts to occur (Fig. 6.2). This is accelerated in women at the time of the menopause and is related to loss of ovarian function (type I osteoporosis). Type II

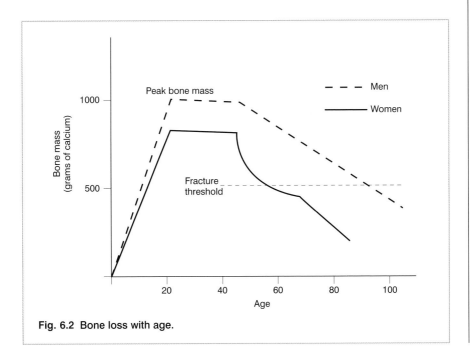

Fig. 6.2 Bone loss with age.

osteoporosis refers to the bone loss that occurs as a consequence of an exaggeration of the normal ageing process.

DIAGNOSIS

To the orthopaedic surgeon fragility fractures represent an end-point problem in osteoporosis demanding technical treatment, which may range from rest, through simple splintage, to internal fixation—or even prosthetic replacement of bone. However, the clinical responsibility of the surgeon does not end with the treatment, but should extend to the exclusion of any underlying metabolic bone disease and the prevention of further fractures at other sites. Inevitably, investigations to detect background bone disease are often overlooked, particularly in patients with fractures of the wrist, humerus, and spine, which require only out-patient treatment. Following a fragility fracture, ideally, all patients should have a biochemical screening of their blood to exclude any metabolic bone disease. Fractures in peri-menopausal women justify referral for measurement of their bone mass, particularly where plain X-ray films suggest the presence of osteoporosis.

Techniques for measuring bone mineral density (BMD)

A large number of techniques have been developed for measuring bone mass. The majority of these use some form of X-ray. The commonest is *Dual Energy X-ray Absorptiometry* (DEXA) scanning. As its name suggests this technique uses X-rays of two different energies. The number of photons that pass through either bone or soft tissue varies according to their energy level. By using two energy levels, it is possible to ascertain the relative degree of absorption by the bone and soft tissues.

This is most commonly used in the more central parts of the skeleton, either the lumbar spine or the femoral neck, but it has also been used peripherally, e.g. in the distal radius. Other techniques include quantitative computed tomography (CT), and ultrasound: several studies have suggested that quantitative ultrasound measurements of the calcaneus are as effective as DEXA scans for predicting the risk of future hip fracture.

Quantitative CT can measure the density of different tissues, provide information on three-dimensional (3D) architecture and in addition can assess the relative contributions of the cancellous and the cortical bone to the total bone density. DEXA, however, is considered to be the gold standard. The BMD correlates well with the bone strength, but it is important to note that BMD only assesses the mineral component of bone and does not assess the 3D architecture of the skeleton, which also has a major bearing on the strength of the bone.

Blood markers

In addition to standard blood measurements of calcium and phosphate levels, it is now possible to measure other parameters that reflect bone formation and resorption. Alkaline phosphatase is an enzyme involved in the mineralisation of bone and osteocalcin is a non-collagenous protein within bone, both of these can be measured in the serum and can be used as indirect indicators of bone formation. Serum markers for bone resorption such as collagen degradation products have been used but found to be less specific indicators of disordered bone metabolism.

RISK FACTORS FOR FRAGILITY FRACTURES

Low bone density (see below)

A decrease in bone density is a major risk factor for a fragility fracture. In addition, a previous fragility factor is also an independent major risk factor for a further fragility fracture.

Falls

If there is a certain risk of fracture each time someone falls onto the floor, then the chance of a person sustaining a fracture depends on: (1) the frequency of falls and (2) the nature of the two objects colliding, i.e. the body and the floor.

Approximately one-third of the elderly population fall annually, the rate is higher in institutionalised individuals and increases with age. It is essential to assess a patient who has had a fragility fracture for their falls risk; it is important to determine if there is any disorder of balance, any postural hypotension and any side effects of medication (Table 6.2) which would predispose the person to falling.

Floor and environment

The hardness of the floor influences the rate of fracture with patients being at higher risk when they fall on a concrete floor compared to a wooden floor. In addition care should be taken to minimise hazards from slippery or uneven floors, poor lighting and electric cables.

Bone strength

This is affected by a number of factors (Table 6.3). Patients who are overweight have a lower risk of fracture. This is due, in part, to a higher BMD but is due also to a degree of cushioning of the fall by the more abundant soft tissues. Bone strength is most commonly assessed by DEXA scans, however, it is important to realise that the levels used to define osteoporosis are to some extent arbitrary and that the fracture risks steadily rise as the BMD falls.

Table 6.2 Drugs affecting the risk of falling

CNS drugs   Benzodiazapines   Antidepressants   Antiepileptic agents
Cardiac drugs   Antihypertensives   Anti-arrhythmics   Diuretics

Table 6.3 Factors affecting bone strength

Age   Gender   Hereditary factors   Age of menarche   Age of menopause   Body weight   Smoking   High alcohol intake

Osteoporosis and fragility fractures

TREATMENT OF OSTEOPOROSIS AND FRACTURE PREVENTION

A number of different modalities are available to the clinician for the treatment of patients following a fragility fracture associated with osteoporosis. The choice of treatment will depend on the age and general health of the patient, as well as their level of activity and social independence. New treatments are continually being introduced in an attempt to reverse this major cause of morbidity in the increasing elderly population with a longer life expectancy.

General measures
All patients should have an adequate intake of calcium (1500 mg/day for the elderly) and vitamin D (400–800 i.u./day), be advised to stop smoking, reduce their alcohol intake and to take regular load-bearing exercise.

Falls prevention strategies
Patients should have a reduction of environmental hazards, appropriate reduction of medication and partake in exercise programmes, such as Tai Chi, to improve muscle strength and balance.

Hip protectors
Hip protectors are padding systems placed over the greater trochanter aimed at shunting or absorbing the energy of the fall away from the bone and thereby preventing fracture. The main problem with them is compliance, with rates of only 25% usage being reported.

Hormone replacement therapy (HRT)
As oestrogen levels fall at the menopause, there is an increase in bone resorption. HRT aims to prevent this increase in resorption. Case controlled studies report a 30% and 50% decrease in hip and spine fractures respectively. However, adverse effects such as an increased risk of DVT, PE and cancer (breast, uterus and ovary) with long-term use have been reported recently and have led to less widespread acceptance of this therapy. HRT may still be of benefit, in patients who have had an early menopause, for a limited treatment period of perhaps several years.

Selective oestrogen receptor modulators (SERMS)
As their name suggests these agents are more selective and can have a positive effect on bone whilst having either no or a negative effect on other tissues such as the endometrium. Raloxifene is one such agent which has been shown to result in a 30–50% reduction in spine fractures; however, the effects on hip fractures were not significant.

Bisphosphonates
The most common drugs used to prevent resorption of bone are the bisphosphonates.

Bisphosphonates are stable analogues of pyrophosphate. They bind strongly to the hydroxyapatite component of bone. They reduce the activity and number of osteoclasts by decreasing their recruitment and increasing their apoptosis. Some patients get temporary 'flu'-like symptoms with their first dose of bisphosphonates and certain foods such as calcium, coffee and tea, reduce the absorption of bisphosphonates such that these drugs need to be taken whilst fasting. The bisphosphonates also can result in dyspepsia, oesophagitis and diarrhoea. However, bisphosphonates have a half life in bone of several years and thus can be administered weekly, monthly or perhaps annually and this helps to reduce the gastrointestinal side effects. Alendronate and risedronate have been reported to reduce hip and spine fractures by approximately 30–50%. However, this effect appears to be primarily in people with a low BMD.

Calcitonin

Calcitonin is a hormone that reduces bone resorption by inhibiting osteoclasts. It can be given subcutaneously, intramuscularly or intranasally. It has been reported to reduce vertebral fractures by approximately 50%.

Bone-forming agents

Currently, agents are under investigation which are thought to have the ability to put the bone back, rather than just prevent its loss, i.e. they may be able to increase bone mass. These include parathyroid hormone and strontium.

Parathyroid hormone (PTH). PTH is the body's main hormone for stimulating bone resorption. Paradoxically when given intermittently it has been shown to increase bone density. It has been reported to result in approximately 70% and 50% reduction of vertebral and non-vertebral fractures respectively. The BMD increased by approximately 10% in the spine and 5% in the femoral neck.

Strontium. Strontium is the newest anti-osteoporosis agent. It is a heavy metal that reduces bone resorption and may like PTH also have an anabolic action on bone. Early results suggest that it may reduce vertebral fractures by 40–50%.

Surgical treatment

It is essential to avoid long-term immobilization, especially in the elderly; as well as inducing bone resorption and muscle wasting these patients are also at risk of pressures sores, chest infections and septicaemia. If fracture treatment is delayed by more than 24 hours, there is an increase in the mortality rate.

In the upper limb the majority of the fragility fractures can be treated non-operatively, although some, such as displaced distal radial fractures may require surgery in order to achieve a good functional outcome.

In the lower limb, in order to achieve early mobilisation the majority require operative treatment. However, the osteoporotic bone in fragility fracture patients poses particular surgical problems and it is much more difficult to get good long-term fixation of the implant with the bone. Devices have been developed such as the 'dynamic hip screw' that allow a degree of sharing of the load between the fracture fragments and the implant. These have resulted in a major drop in the complication rate following hip fracture fixation.

Almost all vertebral fractures used to be treated non-operatively; recently, techniques (vertebroplasty and kyphoplasty) that involve stabilising the vertebral fracture by injecting a material such as bone cement have been used in increased numbers. The benefit of these procedures is still being evaluated.

7 | Joint injuries

In order of decreasing severity, joint injuries may be classed as dislocation, subluxation, strain or contusion.

Before these are described individually it is necessary to consider briefly certain aspects of the normal anatomy of a joint.

The stability of joints

Joint surfaces are held in contact by the shape of the articulating surfaces, by the ligaments, by the surrounding muscles, and by atmospheric pressure. The importance of each of these factors varies with different joints. Thus, in the hip, the deep socket and the almost spherical femoral head, in themselves, afford great security against displacement, and in the elbow also the shape of the bones makes for reasonable intrinsic stability. On the other hand the joints of the fingers, and the knee, depend for their stability mainly on the ligaments, and the shoulder depends largely on the surrounding muscles.

The function of ligaments

The purpose of a ligament is to prevent abnormal movement at a joint. For this it does not always depend entirely on its intrinsic strength; it may rely largely upon the action of the supporting muscles, which contract reflexly to protect the ligament when it comes under harmful stress. Some ligaments are better protected by muscles than others. For example, the ligaments of the shoulder, wrist and hip are well protected by muscles, whereas the collateral ligaments of the finger joints and knee, and the inferior tibio-fibular ligament, are poorly protected. In general, a ligament that is not well guarded by muscles is intrinsically stronger than one that is well protected.

DISLOCATION AND SUBLUXATION

A joint is dislocated or luxated when its articular surfaces are wholly displaced one from the other so that all apposition between them is lost (Figs 7.1C & 7.2). A joint is subluxated when its articular surfaces are partly displaced but retain some contact one with the other (Fig. 7.1B).

Dislocation or subluxation of a joint may be congenital, spontaneous (pathological), traumatic or recurrent. It is only with traumatic and recurrent dislocation or subluxation that we are concerned here.

TRAUMATIC DISLOCATION OR SUBLUXATION

Injury is by far the most common cause of dislocation and subluxation. Any joint may be affected, but those most commonly dislocated are the shoulder, elbow, hip, ankle and interphalangeal joints of the fingers. In many cases

Fig. 7.1 The difference between subluxation and dislocation of a joint. Ⓐ The normal state: joint surfaces congruous. Ⓑ Subluxation: incomplete loss of contact between the joint surfaces. Ⓒ Dislocation: total loss of contact between the joint surfaces.

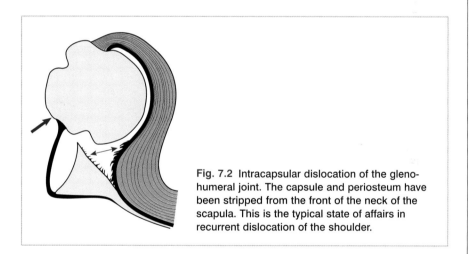

Fig. 7.2 Intracapsular dislocation of the gleno-humeral joint. The capsule and periosteum have been stripped from the front of the neck of the scapula. This is the typical state of affairs in recurrent dislocation of the shoulder.

dislocation or subluxation is associated with a fracture of one or both of the opposing bones: when this occurs the injury is termed a fracture–dislocation or fracture–subluxation.

Dislocation cannot occur without some damage to the protective ligaments and joint capsule. Usually the capsule and one or more of the reinforcing ligaments are torn, permitting the articular end of one of the bones to escape through the rent. Sometimes the capsule is not torn in its substance but is stripped from one of its bony attachments (Fig. 7.2), or, if the ligament withstands the force of the injury, a fragment of bone at one or other attachment of the ligament may be avulsed. It is not always that one of the bone ends protrudes outside the joint capsule; sometimes the joint surfaces may be com-

Joint injuries

Fig. 7.3 A typical anterior (subcoracoid) dislocation of the shoulder.

pletely dislocated and yet both remain within the capsule (intracapsular dislocation, Fig. 7.3).

In joints that depend for their stability mainly upon the surrounding muscles, dislocation will occur most easily when the muscles are off their guard. This probably explains the high incidence of shoulder dislocations in patients suffering epileptic fits.

Diagnosis

In most cases of dislocation the clinical features are sufficiently striking to make the diagnosis obvious. Nevertheless, it not infrequently happens that a dislocation is overlooked, especially when the bony landmarks are obscured by severe swelling or obesity. Certain dislocations are more liable to be overlooked than others: posterior dislocation of the shoulder is particularly notorious in this respect (see Fig. 2.1), and, rather surprisingly, posterior dislocation of the hip is occasionally overlooked when there is a co-existing fracture of the shaft of the femur on the same side.

In doubtful cases, the diagnosis must depend finally on adequate radiographic examination (Fig. 7.3). It must be emphasised that radiographs should always be taken in two planes at right angles to one another, because a dislocation may not be apparent in a single projection (see Fig. 2.1, p. 24). When a dislocation has been reduced, further radiographs should always be obtained to confirm the reduction and determine whether or not there is an associated fracture.

In cases of subluxation the clinical features alone are seldom diagnostic, and reliance must be placed mainly on the radiographic evidence.

As with all limb injuries, specific clinical tests to establish the integrity or otherwise of the major arteries and of the nerves must never be omitted (see p. 21).

Complications

For the most part, the complications that may follow a dislocation are the same as those of a fracture near a joint. They may be summarised as follows:

- infection (after open dislocation)
- injury to important soft-tissue structure (artery, nerve)
- avascular necrosis of one of the articulating bone ends from damage to the vessels supplying it
- persistent instability leading to recurrent dislocation or subluxation
- joint stiffness from intra-articular or peri-articular adhesions, from reflex sympathetic dystrophy or from post-traumatic ossification about the joint ('myositis ossificans')
- osteoarthritis from damage to the articular cartilage or from persistent incongruity of the joint surfaces.

Treatment

Reduction. Clearly the first principle of treatment of a dislocation or subluxation is to reduce the displacement. This is usually achieved by closed manipulation, but sometimes an operation may be required.

Treatment of the ligamentous injury. When the displacement has been corrected the next problem is how to deal with the injury of the soft tissues, and especially of the ligaments. In a few instances a ruptured ligament may be best repaired by operation (for example, a complete rupture of the medial ligament of the knee), but in most cases it may safely be allowed to heal spontaneously. In that case the only remaining question is whether the joint should be immobilised during the stage of healing, or whether movement should be allowed.

It has been found that, in general, normal function is restored most rapidly when movement of the injured joint is encouraged from the beginning or, at the latest, within a few days of the injury. Accordingly, a policy of early mobilisation should be adopted unless special indications for immobilisation exist. Three such indications are: (1) rupture of an important ligament which is largely responsible for the stability of the joint (for example, the conoid and trapezoid ligaments of the acromio-clavicular joint, the medial or lateral ligament of the knee, the lateral ligament of the ankle, and the inferior tibio-fibular ligament); (2) a serious risk of post-traumatic ossification or 'myositis ossificans' (in practice the elbow and possibly the hip are the only joints that need be immobilised on this account); and (3) severe pain.

Treatment of fracture–dislocations. When a dislocation or subluxation is associated with a fracture the principles of treatment are to reduce the joint displacement first, and then to deal with the fracture on its merits.

RECURRENT DISLOCATION OR SUBLUXATION

Certain joints are liable to repeated dislocation or subluxation. Usually, but not always, there has been an initial violent dislocation which leaves the ligaments or the articular surfaces permanently damaged. The joints most often affected are the shoulder (p. 140), sterno-clavicular joint (p. 134), patello-femoral joint (p. 257) and ankle (p. 294).

Joint injuries

STRAIN

A strain is an incomplete rupture of a ligament. It may be acute or chronic.[1] An acute strain is caused by sudden injury, and there is usually macroscopic damage to the ligament. A chronic strain is caused by long-continued stress (for example, foot-strain from prolonged standing), and the changes in the ligament are usually microscopic. We are concerned here only with acute strains.

The force that causes an acute strain is intermediate between one that the ligament can withstand without suffering injury and one that is great enough to rupture the ligament completely. A strain of a ligament that is well protected by muscles may occur either because the force is too great for the muscles to withstand, or because the muscles are caught off their guard.

Clinical features
There is a history of injury such as would impose a stretching force upon the ligament involved. There are local pain and tenderness, with moderate swelling and sometimes a visible ecchymosis. Pain is aggravated when the joint is moved in a direction that tenses the injured ligament.

Diagnosis
Although a strain may be diagnosed with reasonable confidence from the clinical features, radiographs should always be obtained to exclude a fracture or subluxation. In distinguishing between a simple strain and a complete rupture of a ligament, a reliable method is to obtain radiographs while stress is applied to the joint in the direction of the original force, the patient being anaesthetised if necessary. If the ligament is only strained, the joint will remain stable, but if the ligament is torn it will be possible to subluxate the joint, separating the articular surfaces widely on the side of the injury (Figs 7.4 & 15.16B).

It is also significant that an effusion into the joint tends to be more persistent after a strain than after a rupture of a ligament or capsule. This is because in the case of a complete rupture, fluid is able to escape from the joint into the surrounding tissues.

Treatment
The treatment of a strain depends upon the ligament affected and the severity of the pain and disability. As after a dislocation, the general principle should be to encourage early activity and to avoid cumbersome external splintage so far as possible. If pain and swelling are severe it may be wise to immobilise the joint in plaster for the sake of comfort, but immobilisation need never be prolonged for more than 2 or 3 weeks.

---

[1] No sharp distinction is made here between a *strain* and a *sprain*. The term *strain* is preferred, because in technical language it has the meaning that we wish to express, namely structural damage resulting from excessive stress, whereas *sprain* is often used in a lay sense without a precise meaning. Some surgeons, however, restrict the term *strain* to a chronic strain caused by long-continued stress, and use the term *sprain* to denote an acute ligamentous injury.

Fig. 7.4 Doubt about the integrity of a ligament is best resolved by radiographing the joint while the ligament is held under stress by manual force. If the joint space is not shown to be widened on the affected side, the ligament is intact A. Marked widening of the joint space with tilting of the joint surfaces away from one another indicates that the ligament is torn B.

CONTUSION

Contusion of a joint may involve the capsule, synovial membrane and, occasionally, the articular cartilage. The injury sets up a local inflammatory reaction with swelling and serous exudate. *Clinically* there is a history of a direct blow over the joint. There are swelling and local tenderness on palpation. There may be an effusion of fluid in the joint, with slight restriction of movement. Radiographs should always be obtained to exclude the possibility of fracture. Healing occurs spontaneously and only symptomatic treatment is required.

Occasionally, severe contusion of articular cartilage, especially of the hip or metatarso-phalangeal joint of the big toe, has been followed after an interval of months or years by the development of osteoarthritis in the same joint, and a causal relationship must be accepted as probable.

OSTEOCHONDRAL FRACTURE

An injury causing contusion of a joint, if unusually severe, may create an osteochondral fracture. In this injury, probably involving a glancing blow to a convex articular surface, a fragment of cartilage, or of cartilage and sub-chondral bone, may be separated partly or completely from its bed, sometimes forming a loose body within the joint. This injury occurs most commonly in the knee. Because of similar radiographic features this lesion may be confused with osteochondritis dissecans.

8 | Cervical spine

CLASSIFICATION

Injuries of the cervical spine may be classified in two ways, based on the pathological anatomy and on the mechanism that causes the injury.

Pathological anatomy may be classified as follows:

wedge compression fracture of vertebral body p. 97

burst fracture of vertebral body p. 99

extension subluxation p. 99

flexion subluxation p. 99

dislocation and fracture-dislocation p. 100

Cervical spine

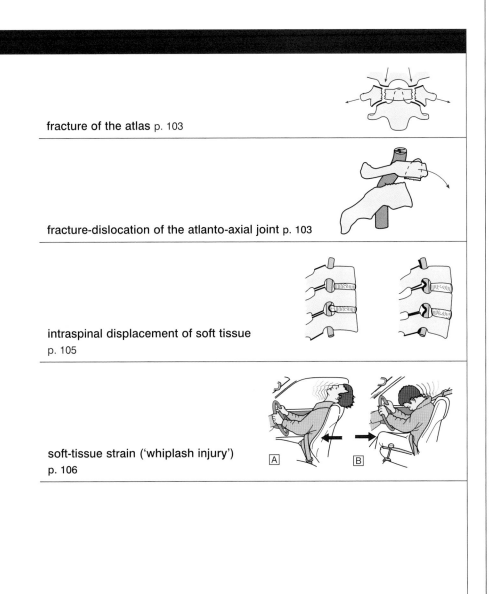

fracture of the atlas p. 103

fracture-dislocation of the atlanto-axial joint p. 103

intraspinal displacement of soft tissue
p. 105

soft-tissue strain ('whiplash injury')
p. 106

Until recently, vertebral injuries were seen less commonly in the cervical spine than in the thoracic and lumbar regions. With the decline in accidents from mining and other heavy industry, and the increase in road traffic accidents, this incidence has changed. Spinal injury units now see as many severe neck injuries as injuries in the rest of the vertebral column. Cervical spine injuries are often more serious, not only on account of a greater risk of injury to the spinal cord, but also because there is a greater liability to persistent disability from aching pain and stiffness of the neck. Moreover, there is an increasing incidence of subluxations and strains in this area caused by sudden recoil of the head in rear-end automobile collisions—the so-called 'whiplash injury'. In most cases the effects are relatively minor from a structural point of view, but disability may, nevertheless, be prolonged.

In many cases violent injuries of the cervical spine cause death so quickly that the patient never reaches the surgeon; thus the cases seen clinically do not reflect the true total incidence of cervical spine injuries.

MECHANISMS THAT COMMONLY RESULT IN INJURY ARE:

flexion
flexion-rotation
extension
vertical compression.

MECHANISM OF INJURY

Major injuries of the cervical spine are usually caused by indirect violence, such as falls onto the head or other violent movements transmitted from the skull. The mechanism may be an excessive movement in any direction—flexion, extension, lateral flexion or rotation—or a vertical compression force acting upon a straight spine. The nature of the injury bears a fairly constant relationship to the mechanism of its causation, but it should be appreciated that many injuries are caused by a combination of forces rather than by violence acting in a single direction.

Flexion and flexion–rotation injuries are common: flexion alone tends to cause a wedge compression fracture (Fig. 8.1A), whereas combined flexion and rotation cause subluxation (Fig. 8.1B), dislocation (Fig. 8.1C) or fracture–dislocation. A flexion or flexion–rotation force may also cause massive displacement of an intervertebral disc, without bone injury (see Fig. 8.13A).

A hyperextension force may fracture the neural arch, especially of the atlas or axis, or it may fracture the dens (odontoid process) of the axis. Alternatively, hyperextension may rupture the anterior longitudinal ligament and the annulus fibrosus, forcing the vertebral bodies apart anteriorly (extension subluxation) (Fig. 8.2). Hyperextension of an osteoarthritic cervical spine, in which the spinal canal is already narrowed by osteophytes, may lead to damage to the spinal cord through impingement upon it of infolded pieces of the tough ligamentum flavum or the osteophytes themselves (Fig. 8.13B); this results in the so-called 'central cord syndrome', with characteristic incomplete loss of neurological function.

Vertical compression acting through the skull may cause a fracture of the ring of the atlas (see Fig. 8.11) or a 'burst' fracture of a vertebral body (Fig. 8.3).

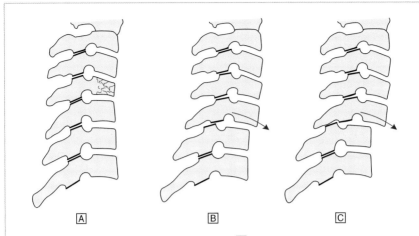

Fig. 8.1 Flexion and flexion-rotation injuries. [A] Wedge compression fracture of a cervical vertebral body. [B] Subluxation of the cervical spine with articular processes dislocation confined to one side. [C] Dislocation of the cervical spine with bilateral articular process dislocation.

Fig. 8.2 Extension subluxation. The anterior longitudinal ligament is ruptured (arrow).

DIAGNOSIS

Cervical injuries are often associated with head injuries, the effects of which may mask the spinal lesion and cause it to be overlooked. It is thus essential that the surgeon take careful note of the condition of the neck (preferably with the help of good radiographs) in every case of serious head injury. An unconscious patient must be assumed to have sustained a neck injury and must be treated accordingly until proved otherwise. Even in the conscious patient, local pain and tenderness in the neck following direct or indirect trauma should be treated as a potential injury to the cervical spine until excluded by imaging.

Fig. 8.3 Burst fracture of vertebral body caused by vertical force acting upon a straight cervical column.

IMAGING

Radiography. Much care is needed in the interpretation of radiographs of the neck. This is often difficult because the cervical vertebrae are irregular in shape, and the shadows of their various processes may be confusing when super-imposed. For this reason it is seldom sufficient to rely only upon antero-posterior and lateral radiographs: additional projections are required. Firstly, lateral radiographs with the head in flexion and extension may reveal instability that is not shown in the routine lateral film. Secondly, oblique views at 45° are especially helpful in demonstrating the intervertebral foramina and the articular processes: they should be taken both from half-right and from half-left because it is not uncommon for subluxation or dislocation of a lateral intervertebral joint to occur on one side only. Thirdly, a special projection through the open mouth (see Fig. 8.12B) is used to obtain an antero-posterior radiograph of the atlas and axis, and in particular of the dens of the axis.

Computed tomography (CT) and magnetic resonance imaging (MRI). The newer imaging techniques of CT and MRI have provided a major advance in the diagnosis of complex spinal injuries. The CT scan provides detailed informa-tion on the bony anatomy, particularly for the identification of small separated fragments or unilateral subluxations (Fig. 8.4A). It has the disadvantage of not providing a rapid screening process for identifying abnormalities in the whole length of the cervical spine, particularly where these affect the soft tissues. MRI, where available, is far more useful for identifying associated soft-tissue injuries, particularly when these involve the spinal cord or nerve roots (Fig. 8.4B). It is the preferred method of imaging whenever there is clinical evidence of spinal cord injury or when herniated intervertebral disc material may have entered the spinal canal.

STABLE AND UNSTABLE INJURIES

It is important to distinguish fractures and dislocations that are stable by virtue of intact posterior ligaments from those that are unstable because the posterior

Fig. 8.4 A Computed tomographic scan of the cervical spine, axial view.
B Magnetic resonance scan of the cervical spine showing a burst fracture (arrow)
of the C4 vertebra with compression of the spinal cord (arrow). (Courtesy of the
Institute of Neurological Sciences, Glasgow.)

ligaments have been torn, usually by a rotation force. A stable fracture or dislocation is not liable to displacement greater than that caused at the time of the injury, whereas an unstable fracture or dislocation is liable to further displacement, with grave peril to the spinal cord. It follows that external splintage or internal fixation may be unnecessary for stable injuries, whereas it is essential for unstable injuries.

WEDGE COMPRESSION FRACTURE OF A VERTEBRAL BODY

A severe flexion force may crush the cancellous bone of one or more of the vertebral bodies (Fig. 8.1A). The compression is always most marked at the front of the vertebral body, which consequently becomes wedge-shaped. The posterior ligaments are intact, so the fracture is stable. This injury is not likely to be complicated by injury to the spinal cord.

Treatment

It is unnecessary to attempt reduction, and all that is required is to support the neck for 2 months to relieve pain. This may be achieved either by a rigid plastic collar (usually of polythene) extending from the chin to the mid-sternum (Fig. 8.5) or, where this is not available, by the use of plaster of Paris. Plastic has the advantage over plaster that the collar may be removed for washing and shaving. When the collar is discarded a course of mobilising and muscle-strengthening exercises should be arranged.

Fig. 8.5 Rigid two-part polythene collar as used for first aid and treatment of minor compression fractures and stable subluxations of the cervical spine.

Ⓐ Ⓑ

Fig. 8.6 Ⓐ Radiograph showing burst fracture of a lower cervical vertebral body. Ⓑ Axial CT scan showing cord compression from posterior displacement of bone fragment.

BURST FRACTURE OF A VERTEBRAL BODY

A 'burst' fracture may be regarded as an uncommon variant of the wedge compression fracture; it is caused by a vertical compression force transmitted directly along the line of the vertebral bodies while the cervical spine is straight, whereas a wedge compression fracture is a consequence of similar violence acting upon a flexed spinal column. The force ruptures one of the vertebral end plates and the intervertebral disc is forced into the body of the vertebra. The effect is to produce a comminuted compression fracture, the fragments of which appear to have burst out peripherally in all directions (Figs 8.3 & 8.6). The spinal cord may escape injury, but often it is damaged by posterior fragments of the vertebral body which may be driven back into it (see Fig. 8.6B). A burst fracture is thus more dangerous than a simple wedge compression fracture. But like the wedge compression fracture it is stable against further displacement because the ligaments are intact.

Treatment

Provided there is no injury to the spinal cord, treatment may be by external support alone. Reduction is not necessary. Sufficient support may be provided by a well-fitted collar of polythene or plaster (Fig. 8.5), as described for wedge compression fracture.

The management of patients with injury to the spinal cord is described in Chapter 10 (p. 122). Whenever possible, such injuries should be treated at a specially equipped centre for paraplegics.

EXTENSION SUBLUXATION

In this uncommon injury the anterior longitudinal ligament is ruptured by a severe extension force and the vertebral bodies are forced apart anteriorly (Fig. 8.2). The spinal cord may or may not escape injury. The spine is unstable in extension but is stable while the neck is in the neutral position or in flexion.

Treatment

The neck must be supported in the neutral position or in slight flexion, preferably by a rigid plastic collar which should be retained for at least 2 months.

FLEXION SUBLUXATION

In flexion subluxation of the cervical spine there is forward displacement of one vertebra upon another, but the displacement is not sufficient to cause total overriding of the articular processes (Figs 8.1B & 8.7). Often there is a rotational element in the causative violence, with the consequence that overriding of the articular processes, either partial or complete, occurs on one side only (Fig. 8.7). The injury usually occurs in the lower half of the cervical column. It is frequently missed because the displacement between the vertebral bodies, as seen in the lateral radiograph, may be slight or absent.

Clinically, there is severe pain and the patient is unwilling to move the neck. Radiographs usually confirm the diagnosis when there has been a unilateral facet dislocation or fracture causing a slight but characteristic (25%) displacement of the upper vertebral body upon the lower (Fig. 8.7). In cases of doubt, oblique radiographs will confirm displacement or fracture of the facet on one side but not on the other. In some cases of subluxation the displacement may

Fig. 8.7 Minor anterior subluxation of a cervical vertebral body associated with unilateral facet dislocation.

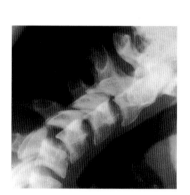

Fig. 8.8 Marked forward displacement of a cervical vertebral body with bilateral facet dislocation.

be corrected spontaneously when the head is held erect, and the injury may thus be overlooked unless radiographs are taken with the neck slightly flexed. Since the posterior ligaments are damaged the injury must be regarded as unstable.

In cases of subluxation the spinal cord usually escapes serious injury, but if the spine is affected by osteoarthritis even slight subluxation may be dangerous, because the spinal canal may already be narrowed by osteophytes.

Treatment

It is necessary first to reduce the subluxation and thereafter to prevent redisplacement by holding the neck extended. If the subluxation is reduced simply by extending the neck, as is often the case, splintage alone may be all that is required to prevent redisplacement. Splintage must be designed to prevent flexion of the neck, and it may be achieved either by a rigid plastic collar moulded well down over the sternum, or by an adjustable 'four-poster' splint. When displacement of one facet has occurred, skull traction may be required to achieve reduction, and it may need to be continued for 4 weeks or so while early healing of the soft tissues occurs. Thereafter it may be replaced by a suitable splint. In all cases support should be maintained for 2 months from the time of injury.

Vertebrae that have been displaced often become stabilised spontaneously by the formation of a buttress of bone anteriorly. However, if follow-up radiographs show that the cervical spine continues to subluxate in flexion, local fusion of the affected vertebrae by posterior wiring and bone grafting should be advised.

DISLOCATION AND FRACTURE–DISLOCATION

The articular surfaces are out of contact and there is overriding of the articular processes (Figs 8.1C & 8.8). There may be associated compression fractures of the vertebral bodies or a fracture of the neural arch. This is a very unstable injury.

Damage to the spinal cord—often complete transection but sometimes an incomplete lesion—is a common complication of this injury. Nevertheless, it is surprising what severe displacement may sometimes occur without injury to the spinal cord.

Treatment

Careful handling is necessary lest further displacement cause or aggravate an injury of the spinal cord. Flexion of the neck must be avoided.

Reduction is best effected by skull traction under radiographic control. Traction is applied through skull calipers, the tips of which engage in small holes through the outer table of the skull only, made low in each parietal region (Fig. 8.9). With this method, traction of up to 20 pounds (9 kg) can be maintained without much discomfort to the patient, and this is often sufficient to disengage the overriding articular processes within a few hours. While this heavy traction is being applied it is important that a close watch be kept on the patient's neurological state, because it is possible to damage the spinal cord or the medulla by injudicious traction on an injured spine. When radiographs confirm that the articular processes have been disengaged, reduction is completed by gradually extending the cervical spine. Light traction is then maintained for 3 weeks if there seems any risk of redisplacement. Alternatively, earlier mobilisation may be permitted in the absence of paraplegia by the application of a 'halo' splint (Fig. 8.10). This provides far greater stability than a conventional polythene or plaster of Paris collar, which should only be used in the later stages of treatment when soft-tissue healing is advanced.

Fig. 8.9 Cone's (Barton's) traction calipers applied to a skull to show the position of insertion of the points.

Cervical spine

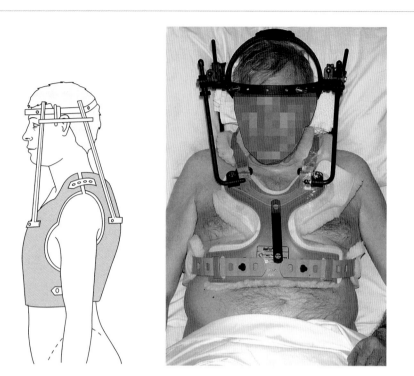

Fig. 8.10 Halo-thoracic support. The halo—a metal ring—is screwed to the skull, and vertical struts unite it to a plastic thoracic vest or to a body plaster. This device gives better immobilisation of the cervical spine than any other splint.

Indications for operation
Operation may be required for: (1) irreducible locking of articular processes and (2) persistent instability.

Irreducible locking of articular processes. If interlocked articular processes cannot be disengaged by traction, operative excision of the processes obstructing reduction may be necessary. This is most likely to be the case when attempted reduction has been delayed for more than 1 week. Operative reduction should be followed by posterior fusion of the affected segments of the spine by means of wiring and bone grafts.

Persistent instability. If gradual redisplacement occurs after initial reduction and immobilisation, it may be advisable to stabilise the affected region of the spine by operative fusion. The operation entails the placing of bone grafts to bridge the joint below the displaced vertebra. In posterior fusion the grafts are placed between the spinous processes and laminae; at the same time the spinous processes are wired together with stainless-steel wire to ensure fixation while the bone grafts become incorporated. Alternatively, fusion may be secured anteriorly by laying a bone graft in a deep slot cut in the front of the bodies of the affected vertebrae.

In many cases stabilisation of the affected segments of the spinal column occurs spontaneously through the formation of a buttress of bone beneath the previously unstable vertebral body, thus obviating the need for operative stabilisation. Accordingly, it may be appropriate to advise a period of observation before a decision is made on whether operative fusion should be undertaken.

Spinal cord injury

The management of patients with tetraplegia or paraplegia is considered separately in Chapter 10 (p. 122).

FRACTURE OF THE ATLAS

The atlas may be fractured by vertical force acting through the skull, the bony ring formed by the anterior arch and the posterior arch of the atlas being forced open by the impact of the occipital condyles (Fig. 8.11). It corresponds to the burst fracture already described for the lower cervical vertebrae (p. 99). Displacement is seldom severe, and more often than not the spinal cord escapes serious injury.

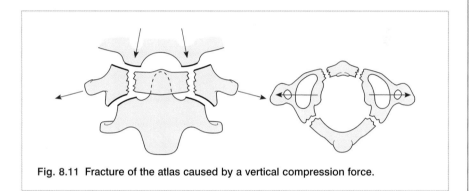

Fig. 8.11 Fracture of the atlas caused by a vertical compression force.

Treatment

In the absence of injury to the spinal cord it is sufficient to support the injured region for 3 months by a plaster or plastic collar (Fig. 8.5), or by a halo-thoracic support (Fig. 8.10).

FRACTURE–DISLOCATION OF THE ATLANTO-AXIAL JOINT(Fracture of the dens of the axis)

The normal atlanto-axial joint depends for its stability upon the snug fit of the anterior arch and the transverse ligament of the atlas over the dens (odontoid process) of the axis. This stability may be lost if the transverse ligament is defective or if the dens is fractured. Forward displacement of the atlas from inflammatory softening of the transverse ligament is well recognised in cases of infection involving the throat or neck, but traumatic rupture of the ligament is seldom seen clinically. When the atlas is displaced by violence there is nearly always a fracture at the base of the dens, and the dens fragment is displaced together with the atlas. Displacement is forwards in flexion injuries (Fig. 8.12A), and backwards in extension injuries. Forward displacement is the more common. Sometimes there is a fracture of the dens without displacement.

Fig. 8.12 Ⓐ Lateral radiograph showing atlanto-axial dislocation due to fracture of the base of the dens. The spinal cord often escapes serious damage. Ⓑ 'Open mouth' radiographic projection showing fracture of base of dens.

It is difficult to assess the true incidence of injury to the spinal cord from fracture–dislocation of the atlanto-axial joint, because complete transection of the cord at this level would cause immediate death and the patient would not reach the surgeon. In the cases seen clinically, however, there is usually either no evidence of spinal cord damage or only slight dysfunction. Sometimes there has been late paresis from gradual secondary displacement of an ununited fracture.

Clinically, patients are often seen supporting their head in their hands. Diagnosis depends upon radiological examination (p. 96), which must include an 'open mouth' view (Fig. 8.12B).

Treatment

If there is no displacement it is sufficient to immobilise the cervical spine and occiput for 10–12 weeks. The fullest immobilisation is provided by a halo-cast, the term used for a metal ring or 'halo' screwed to the skull, with vertical struts incorporated in a body cast or plastic vest enclosing the thoracic region (Fig. 8.10). Alternatively, an extensive plaster jacket extended upwards to grip the skull (Minerva jacket) may be used. If severe displacement is present it must be reduced either by gentle manipulation or by skull traction before a halo-cast is applied.

Bony union does not always occur but close fibrous union is usually adequate. Occasionally, persistent instability demands local operative fusion between the atlas and axis.

INTRASPINAL DISPLACEMENT OF SOFT TISSUE

Rarely, cases of neck injury are encountered in which there has clearly been a severe injury to the spinal cord—as evidenced by partial or complete tetraplegia or paraplegia—and yet there is no radiographic sign of bone injury or displacement. In some such cases it is possible that the cord injury has been caused by momentary vertebral displacement that has become reduced spontaneously (Fig. 8.2). In other instances, however, it has been shown that forcible displacement of soft tissue into the spinal canal has been responsible. The soft tissue concerned may be: (1) the nucleus pulposus of an intervertebral disc or (2) a posterior fold of ligamentum flavum.

Displacement of intervertebral disc material

Massive prolapse of the nucleus pulposus of an intervertebral disc is a well-recognised cause of spinal cord compression (Fig. 8.13A). When the prolapse occurs suddenly from injury, a violent flexion–compression force is usually responsible. The displacement may be demonstrated by myelography or CT scanning, and if the cord is not irreparably damaged, relief may follow operative removal of the displaced disc material.

Infolding of ligamentum flavum

It has been shown that in full extension of the cervical spine, folds of the ligamentum flavum become invaginated into the spinal canal, and these

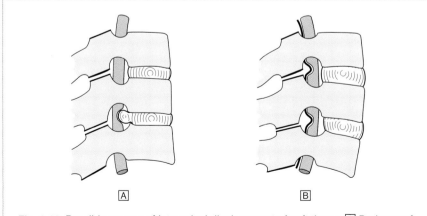

Fig. 8.13 Possible causes of intraspinal displacement of soft tissue. A Prolapse of intervertebral disc. B Infolding of ligamentum flavum.

indentations, if produced suddenly by a hyperextension injury, may be sufficient to damage the spinal cord (Fig. 8.13B). The risk of cord injury from this cause is greatly increased if the spinal canal is already narrowed by the encroachment of osteophytes in a patient with advanced osteoarthritis, which may also lead to ossification of the infolded ligaments. The patient may show bruising of the face, an indication that a hyperextension injury has occurred. Contusion at the centre of the spinal cord causes the characteristic features of the 'central cord syndrome'. There is usually almost complete motor paralysis distal to the level of the lesion, but with preservation of some sensory function. Some recovery of motor power may be expected, but in only about half the cases is it sufficient to permit walking without support.

SOFT-TISSUE STRAIN OF THE CERVICAL SPINE ('WHIPLASH' INJURY)

Soft-tissue strain of the cervical spine—often termed 'whiplash injury'—is common in occupants of cars struck violently from behind by other vehicles ('rear-end shunts').

Mechanism of injury and pathology

At the moment of impact, the head is first thrown backwards as the vehicle is suddenly jolted forwards (Fig. 8.14A). This is followed by rebound flexion of the neck, (Fig. 8.14B) often so extreme that the chin abuts against the chest, and by a second extension movement. It is assumed that there is strain of the deep muscles and ligaments of the cervical spine. If the head happens to be rotated at the moment when the collision occurs, as is often the case, there is also strain of the lateral muscles (mainly the trapezius) on the side to which the head is turned. In theory, a force of extreme violence could cause immediate death from major fracture–dislocation of the cervical spine, but such cases are

Fig. 8.14 Mechanism of 'Whiplash injury' A Extension force at impact. B Rebound flexion of the neck.

unlikely to be seen clinically. In the great majority of cases, radiographs do not show any structural damage in the spinal column.

Clinical features

At impact, the patient may feel jolting or 'wrenching' of the neck or of one or other shoulder, but often there is no severe pain initially and the patient may think at first that he or she has escaped significant injury. However, within hours of the accident—occasionally as late as a day or more afterwards—there is increasing pain and 'stiffness' in the back of the neck, often with extension to the top and back of one or other shoulder. The neck pain is usually accompanied by severe headache, which may be persistent and which may possibly result from a jarring motion of the brain within the skull at the time of the to-and-fro movement of the head. Examination shows restriction of the range of movement of the cervical spine, usually in all directions at first, but later more localised. If pain extends to one or other shoulder there is also slight restriction of elevation and medial rotation of the arm, but other movements are free and there is nothing to suggest that there has been damage to the shoulder joint itself.

Symptoms from whiplash injury of the neck are often very slow to subside and, whereas some patients show full recovery in a matter of weeks, it is common for patients to complain of lingering neck and shoulder pain, with or without frequent headache, for as long as 1 or 2 years and sometimes for even longer. In long-protracted cases it is often found that the patient has become demoralised, and psychological factors may delay recovery.

Treatment

The condition does not respond well to any particular form of treatment: as is so often the case with soft-tissue strains, time is the best healer. In general, the principle of treatment should be to provide support and rest for the neck at first, in the form of a protective cervical collar. But after 1 or 2 weeks the emphasis should be on the restoration of mobility by exercises within the limits imposed by pain, preferably under the supervision of a physiotherapist. Many patients also resort to osteopathy, which is not harmful if treatment is confined to local massage, gentle manipulation and encouragement in exercises. Forcible manipulation is, however, to be avoided.

9 | Spine and thorax

CLASSIFICATION

Injuries of the spine and thorax may be classified as follows:

Major fractures and displacements of the thoracic or lumbar vertebrae.

Wedge compression fracture of a vertebral body p. 111

Burst fracture of a vertebral body p. 115

Distraction fracture of a vertebral body p. 116

Dislocation and fracture-dislocation p. 117

Minor fractures of the spinal column.
Fractures of transverse processes
Fracture of the sacrum
Fracture of the coccyx

Fractures of the thoracic cage.
Fractures of the ribs
Fractures of the sternum

Fractures at any level in the spine may involve the vertebral bodies or the posterior elements—transverse processes and spinous processes. Injuries of the vertebral bodies tend to occur from compression, flexion or twisting forces, whereas the posterior elements are more likely to be damaged by direct violence.

Many spinal injuries are benign and cause little or no permanent disability. The important exception, of course, is a major vertebral fracture or displacement in which the spinal cord or cauda equina is damaged. These are grave injuries, often resulting in permanent paralysis. Nevertheless, the more aggressive approach that is now being widely advocated has given encouraging results in a proportion of cases in which the neural injury has been incomplete.

Fractures of the thoracic cage may be relatively minor injuries, as for instance when a single rib is fractured, but chest injuries must never be regarded lightly because complications are common and often serious. Indeed, a major crushing injury of the chest is one of the most lethal emergencies in the whole realm of accident surgery.

MAJOR FRACTURES AND DISPLACEMENTS OF THE THORACIC AND LUMBAR VERTEBRAE

These are the most common spinal fractures seen in clinical practice and they demand detailed consideration.

MECHANISM OF INJURY

Fractures of the thoracic or lumbar vertebral bodies are nearly always caused by vertical force acting through the long axis of the spinal column. This force may act from above, as when a coal miner is buried by a fall of roof, or from below, as by a heavy fall on the feet or buttocks, in high speed motor vehicle collisions, or in the emergency use of an aircraft ejection seat. The thoraco-lumbar junction is most vulnerable as the upper thoracic vertebrae are protected by the bracing effect of the rib cage. Since the natural curve of the spine is predominantly one of flexion, the effect of such a force is to increase the flexion (Fig. 9.1). Accordingly, it is found that most vertebral fractures in the thoracic or thoraco-lumbar region are hyperflexion injuries and that fractures from hyperextension are uncommon. If the affected part of the spinal column is straight at the moment of impact the compression force, acting directly along the line of the vertebral bodies, may cause a 'burst' fracture like that described in the cervical region (p. 97).

In the usual flexion injury one or more of the vertebral bodies collapses anteriorly and becomes wedge-shaped, giving rise to a localised kyphosis (Fig. 9.2). This is the common wedge compression fracture of a vertebral body.

When the causative violence is very severe high-energy trauma, and especially if the flexion force is accompanied by rotation or distraction, fracture of a vertebral body may be complicated by dislocation of the adjacent intervertebral joint, with forward displacement of the upper vertebra upon the lower (Figs 9.3 & 9.4). This is the dangerous condition of fracture–dislocation of the spine, which is so often complicated by damage to the spinal cord or cauda equina and consequent paralysis.

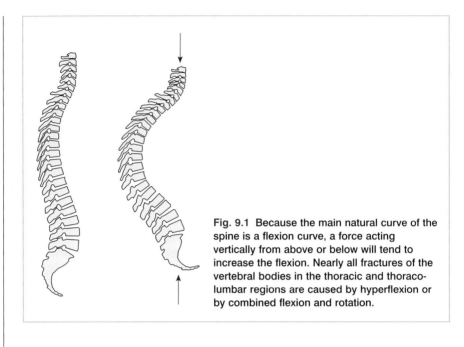

Fig. 9.1 Because the main natural curve of the spine is a flexion curve, a force acting vertically from above or below will tend to increase the flexion. Nearly all fractures of the vertebral bodies in the thoracic and thoraco-lumbar regions are caused by hyperflexion or by combined flexion and rotation.

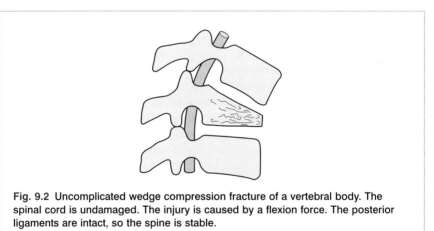

Fig. 9.2 Uncomplicated wedge compression fracture of a vertebral body. The spinal cord is undamaged. The injury is caused by a flexion force. The posterior ligaments are intact, so the spine is stable.

STABLE AND UNSTABLE INJURIES

As in the case of cervical injuries (p. 96), it is important to distinguish between fractures and fracture–dislocations in which intact posterior ligaments make the spine stable against further displacement, and those unstable injuries in which rupture of the posterior ligaments might permit further displacement, with peril to the spinal cord or cauda equina. The distinction is fundamental from the point of view of treatment, because a spine that is stable does not necessarily require protection whereas an unstable spine must be protected either by external support or by internal fixation.

Fig. 9.3 Vertebral fracture–dislocation with transection of the spinal cord. Note the characteristic slice fracture of the vertebral body. The injury is caused by combined flexion and rotation.

Ⓐ   Ⓑ

Fig. 9.4 Ⓐ CT scan of thoraco-lumbar dislocation. Ⓑ A fracture–dislocation in which the lower end of the spinal cord was crushed.

WEDGE COMPRESSION FRACTURE OF A VERTEBRAL BODY

Diagnosis

In cases of major fracture there will be obvious symptoms and signs pointing to an injury of the spinal column, most commonly between the T11 and L2 vertebrae. It should be remembered, however, that the symptoms and signs of a simple compression fracture are often surprisingly slight; they may be overlooked by patient and doctor alike, especially if more painful injuries to other parts of the body are also present. Careful enquiry and examination should therefore be made to determine the presence or absence of the following features that suggest fracture: local pain; a prominent spinous process on palpation; tenderness on percussion; and painful limitation of spinal movement. In some cases a spinal fracture may simulate an intra-abdominal lesion, and the abdomen may be opened injudiciously in a fruitless search for a ruptured viscus if the real cause of the symptoms is overlooked. The possibility of a vertebral fracture should always be borne in mind in cases of violent injury, and it is worth remembering that a considerable proportion of cases of crush fracture of the calcaneus (an injury that is usually caused by a fall from a height on to the heels) are associated with compression fracture of the spine. If there is any doubt about the possibility of a spinal fracture, radiographs must always be obtained, because if a fracture is overlooked and left untreated there is a possibility of persistent back pain later.

Most wedge compression fractures are inherently stable because the posterior structures are intact. Instability should always be suspected if wedging of a vertebral body is associated with a 'slice' fracture (Fig. 9.3), because this indicates that the injury has been one of combined flexion and rotation. There may be unilateral fracture or subluxation of a facet joint, which may be revealed only on oblique radiographs or computed tomographic (CT) scans. Such an injury is important because it may be complicated by later vertebral displacement.

It should be remembered that the spinal column is a common site for pathological fractures, particularly in the older patient with osteoporosis or metastatic tumour (Fig. 9.5). Crush fracture of the vertebral body in osteoporosis is the commonest of the fragility fractures associated with this condition. Its onset may be associated with an episode of minor trauma, but is frequently insidious without significant injury and with only minor local pain. More commonly, the patient presents with progressive loss of height and an increasing kyphotic deformity of the thoracic spine, the so-called 'dowager's hump'. This results from collapse of the thoracic vertebrae at several levels with anterior wedging of the bodies. In advanced cases the radiographs show little difference between the density of the bone and the intervertebral discs, which characteristically show bulging into the weakened bodies, particularly in the lumbar spine (Fig. 9.5A).

Treatment

It has been shown that persistent wedging of a vertebral body is compatible with virtually normal function, so correction of the deformity is not essential. The standard method of treatment may, therefore, be said to be conservative, though some prefer an interventionist approach.

Standard method. The standard method of treatment in a case of moderate severity is to nurse the patient free in bed in the early stages and to concentrate entirely on restoring function. To this end active muscle exercises, mainly for the erector spinae muscles, are begun immediately and are intensified progressively as the pain subsides. The patient is allowed up as soon as pain permits (usually 1–3 weeks after the injury), and thereafter rehabilitation is continued under the supervision of a skilled physiotherapist by exercises designed both to strengthen the spinal muscles and to restore mobility.

Fig. 9.5 The spinal column is a common site for pathological fractures. The two most common causes are senile osteoporosis Ⓐ and metastatic carcinomatous deposits Ⓑ.

In a small proportion of wedge fractures of a vertebral body, the severity of pain may justify the use of a thoraco-lumbar spinal brace, which will often facilitate earlier mobilisation and limit excessive flexion during the healing period.

Osteoporotic fragility fracture. Until recently, treatment of this disabling condition was confined to symptomatic pain medication and re-assurance. Greater awareness of the morbidity of the fracture in a rapidly increasing elderly population with greater longevity has led to more active medical and surgical interventions. As outlined in Chapter 6 (p. 82), all patients should be investigated to determine the cause and extent of their bone loss and, where appropriate, medical treatment instituted to prevent further progression. In selected cases where local pain is more severe and of recent onset, a new minimally invasive surgical treatment of balloon kyphoplasty may be considered. The technique is still under trial and is only available in specialised centres, as it requires sophisticated imaging support. A percutaneous probe is inserted, using radiographic screening, into the centre of the collapsed vertebral body and is then replaced with a bone tamp. This balloon-like device is then inflated with contrast medium until the vertebral body height is restored. Finally, the space is injected with semi-liquid polymethylmethacrylate cement, which, once solidified, will restore the vertebral bone stability.

Alternative methods for special cases. Conservative treatment is appropriate and adequate for most wedge fractures, but when loss of vertebral body height exceeds 50%, or the kyphosis exceeds 30°, the posterior ligamentous structures are probably disrupted and justify operative intervention. Posterior stabilisation and indirect reduction by distraction are usually used and will achieve some correction of deformity as well as facilitating the patient's rehabilitation. In severe fracture dislocation, fixation may be achieved by the use of posterior instrumentation using a metal Hartshill rectangle (Fig. 9.6) or Luque rods, which lie posteriorly and are wired to the laminae of each vertebra in the region to be stabilised. Both these devices have the disadvantage of extending over several non-affected spinal segments. Recently, there has been an increasing use of pedicle screw fixation devices, consisting of shorter rods anchored by screws inserted into the vertebral bodies through the pedicles (Fig. 9.7).

Fig. 9.6 Fixation of L1/L2 dislocation by posterior rectangle held by sublaminal wiring.

Fig. 9.7 Unstable thoraco-lumbar fracture dislocation after pedicle screw fixation.

BURST FRACTURE OF A VERTEBRAL BODY

This is a less common variant of the wedge compression fracture in which the spine is straight at the moment of injury: the compression force thus acts vertically in the line of the vertebral bodies. The intervertebral disc is forced into the affected vertebral body, causing a comminuted bursting fracture in which fragments are driven outwards in all directions. Posterior fragments may be driven into the spinal cord or cauda equina; so this injury must be regarded as much more dangerous than the simple wedge compression fracture (Fig. 9.8).

In this type of injury, CT scanning or magnetic resonance scanning should be undertaken to show to what extent, if any, bone fragments are encroaching upon the spinal canal (Fig. 10.1, p. 123).

Treatment

This fracture must be regarded as less stable than a simple compression fracture. If there is no neurological impairment, it is permissible to employ conservative treatment as for wedge compression fracture, but a rather longer period of recumbency is advisable. An increasing number of surgeons now tend to favour internal fixation (see previous section), and there are some who would advocate a decompressive operation to remove fragments that encroach on the spinal canal even in the absence of neurological deficit. The treatment of fractures complicated by nerve damage is discussed in the next chapter (p. 126).

Fig. 9.8 A Radiograph and B CT scan of L1 burst fractures showing backward displacement of bony fragment into the spinal canal.

DISTRACTION FRACTURE OF A VERTEBRAL BODY

This is another uncommon fracture, which usually occurs in the L1 vertebra and is often missed in the initial radiographic assessment. The causation is a high-velocity hyperflexion force applied to the upper trunk when the pelvis and lower spine are restrained. It was more common in motor vehicle accidents when only lap seatbelts were used, without the addition of a shoulder strap. This provided an anterior fulcrum for the high-energy deceleration force to distract the posterior structures. Radiographs appear to show a compression fracture of the body, but the fracture gap can be seen to extend posteriorly through the pedicle and lamina at the same level, making it a potentially unstable injury (Fig. 9.9).

Treatment

Despite the severity of this injury, there is a low incidence of associated neurological impairment, though if CT scanning confirms an unstable fracture, it should be stabilised with posterior instrumentation to prevent any risk of secondary damage. Because of the mechanism of the injury, there is a high incidence (40–50%) of associated intra-abdominal visceral damage requiring careful patient examination and monitoring in the post-injury period.

Fig. 9.9 Ⓐ Lateral radiograph and Ⓑ CT scan of distraction fracture of L1 vertebra.

DISLOCATION AND FRACTURE–DISLOCATION

These injuries are uncommon compared with simple wedge compression fractures of the vertebral bodies.

The most common displaced injury of the thoracic or lumbar spine is a fracture–dislocation, in which one of the vertebrae is forced forwards upon the vertebra next below it (Figs 9.3 & 9.4). This can occur only if the articular processes are fractured, or if the facet joints are dislocated and the articular processes overridden. At the same time the lower of the two affected vertebral bodies is fractured near its upper surface: typically the fracture line is almost horizontal, giving the appearance in the radiograph that the vertebra has been sliced (Fig. 9.3). The posterior ligaments are always torn, so the spine is very unstable and further displacement may easily occur. Most of these fracture–dislocations occur in the mid-thoracic region or at the thoraco-lumbar junction (Fig. 9.6), and it has been shown that the causative violence is nearly always a combined flexion and rotation force.

Fracture–dislocation in the thoracic region or at the thoraco-lumbar junction is nearly always complicated by injury to the spinal cord, and the cord injury is usually a complete transection. Fracture–dislocation in the lumbar region is often complicated by injury to the cauda equina, which may be complete or incomplete.

Treatment

In most of these injuries, paraplegia from injury to the spinal cord overshadows the skeletal injury. The management of such cases is considered separately in the chapter on paraplegia (Chapter 10, p. 122).

In the occasional case in which a fracture–dislocation or a dislocation is not complicated by paraplegia, the patient must be handled with great care lest further vertebral displacement should injure the spinal cord. Flexion and extension of the spine should both be avoided while the patient is transported, preferably on a spineboard, and the injury is fully assessed radiologically.

Though reduction of the displacement by posture and traction may be practicable, most surgeons would now favour operative reduction and internal fixation by Harrington rods, Luque rods, or pedicle screw fixation.

MINOR FRACTURES OF THE SPINAL COLUMN

Minor fractures of the vertebrae are mainly fractures of the transverse processes, undisplaced fractures of the sacrum and fractures of the coccyx. These injuries are referred to as minor fractures because they are not likely to be complicated by catastrophes such as spinal cord injury and because, if treated efficiently, they do not lead to permanent disability. On the other hand, they can be very painful injuries, and they demand careful nursing and energetic physical treatment like the more serious fractures.

FRACTURES OF TRANSVERSE PROCESSES

These injuries are almost confined to the lumbar region. They are caused by direct violence such as a heavy blow or a fall against a hard object. The injury may involve a single transverse process, but often two or more processes are fractured on the same side (Fig. 9.10). Occasionally, there may be associated damage to the corresponding kidney or to the spleen.

Fig. 9.10 Fractures of the fourth and fifth left lumbar transverse processes.

Treatment

Treatment starts with rest in bed until the acute pain subsides. At an early stage active exercises for the spinal muscles are begun and are intensified as the pain becomes less. After a few days or 1 week, according to progress, the patient begins to get up, but should continue an active programme of rehabilitation until full function has been regained.

FRACTURE OF THE SACRUM

This uncommon injury is caused by a fall or direct blow on the sacral region. The fracture is usually no more than a crack without displacement. It may be suspected clinically from the presence of marked local tenderness, and later from the appearance of an ecchymosis. In the absence of complications no special treatment is required.

Displaced fractures. In the rare instances in which the fragments are markedly displaced, there is a serious risk of injury of the cauda equina or of component nerves of the sacral plexus.

FRACTURE OF THE COCCYX

A fracture of the coccyx may be caused by a fall on the 'tail'. It is an uncommon injury. In nearly every circumstance the pain will subside gradually without special treatment, but in the exceptional case in which pain from an ununited fracture persists for many months, the coccyx may be excised.

FRACTURES OF THE THORACIC CAGE

FRACTURES OF THE RIBS

Most fractures of the ribs are caused by direct injury, as by a fall against a hard object. Occasionally, a rib may be fractured by laughing or coughing, when the bone is weakened by severe osteoporosis or metastases.

The fracture usually occurs near the angle of the rib. There is seldom severe displacement, because the fragments are held well together by the attached muscles. In the event of marked displacement, or when there are multiple rib fractures, a fragment may pierce the pleura or lung, with consequent haemothorax or haemopneumothorax.

Clinical features

There is severe pain made worse by deep breathing, with marked local tenderness on palpation over the site of fracture. Antero-posterior compression of the thorax by springing the ribs also causes pain at the site of fracture. The diagnosis is confirmed by radiography.

Treatment

Fractures of the ribs unite spontaneously, and treatment is required only to increase the patient's comfort and to combat possible complications. Breathing exercises should be encouraged to ensure that the lung is fully expanded. In severe cases pain may be relieved by injecting a solution of long-acting local anaesthetic about the site of fracture.

Complications

The main importance of fractures of the ribs is that they may give rise to pulmonary complications that may sometimes be serious or even fatal in the absence of prompt and efficient treatment. The complications include haemothorax, pneumothorax, surgical emphysema and pneumonia. As one might expect, they are most common after violent direct injuries, and they are liable to be especially serious in elderly patients with multiple rib fractures. Treatment is outlined below.

FRACTURES OF THE STERNUM

A fracture of the sternum may be caused in two ways: (1) by direct injury or (2) by vertical compression of the thoracic cage, with simultaneous fracture of the thoracic spine.

Fractures from direct injury are seen rather commonly in drivers after collision with another vehicle, with impact of the front of the chest against the steering wheel. In most cases the injury is no more than a crack fracture, but it is associated with severe pain. In more violent injuries the sternum is driven in from the front, reducing the antero-posterior diameter of the thorax and impairing the vital capacity. If displacement is marked it should be corrected by open surgical reduction.

Sternal fractures associated with compression fracture of the thoracic spine are well recognised but uncommon. The spinal injury is caused in the usual way by hyperflexion, and the force is transmitted to the sternum through the ribs. The sternum is angled backwards at the fracture, which occurs near the

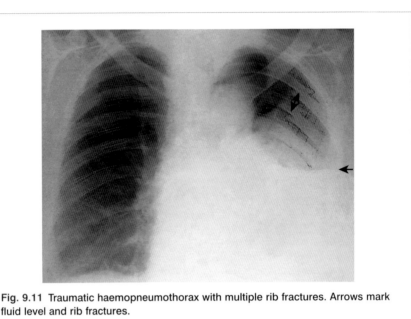

Fig. 9.11 Traumatic haemopneumothorax with multiple rib fractures. Arrows mark fluid level and rib fractures.

junction of the manubrium and the body of the sternum, but displacement is seldom severe. Treatment is required mainly for the associated fracture of the spine. No special treatment is needed for the sternal fracture.

PRINCIPLES OF TREATMENT OF MAJOR CHEST INJURIES

In cases of severe injury to the thoracic cage, and especially when multiple rib fractures on both sides create a flail anterior segment of chest wall ('stove-in chest') (Fig. 9.11), prompt treatment may be required to save life.

The danger arises from the patient's inability to take proper breaths on account of obstruction of the airway, filling of the pleural cavity by blood or air, loss of rigidity of the thoracic cage with consequent paradoxical respiration, severe pain, or a combination of several or all of these hindrances. Clearly, treatment must be designed to correct or counteract any condition that is preventing adequate respiration. In the worst emergencies, with the patient badly cyanosed and showing paradoxical respiration, he or she should be anaesthetised forthwith to allow respiration to be controlled mechanically while the necessary action is taken.

Airway. It may be necessary repeatedly to remove bronchial secretions by suction. This is facilitated by tracheostomy. Tracheostomy also aids oxygenation by reducing the dead-space air, and it permits long-term mechanical control of respiration when this is required. On the other hand it is unpleasant for the patient and should not be performed needlessly.

Pleural drainage. Respiratory embarrassment by blood or air in the pleural cavity is corrected by drainage through a tube inserted through an upper intercostal space and led to a suction bottle. Pleural drainage is required as an emergency procedure in cases of tension pneumothorax.

Flail anterior segment of chest wall. If the necessary equipment and staff are available, paradoxical respiration from multiple rib fractures with flail anterior segment is best controlled by intermittent positive pressure respiration with a mechanical respirator. Otherwise, steps may have to be taken to fix fractures of the sternum and ribs by stiff intramedullary wires, in order to restore rigidity to the thoracic cage.

Pain. In cases of moderate severity, pain may be controlled adequately by appropriate drugs and by injection of a long-acting local anaesthetic solution about the fractures. In the worst cases there is a place for long-term inhalation anaesthesia or continuous epidural block.

10 Paraplegia from spinal injuries

Damage to the spinal cord or cauda equina complicates between 10 and 20% of all spinal injuries. Most of these injuries occur in a younger 16–30 year age group, with an increasing incidence due to motor vehicle accidents. An increasing number result from sporting accidents, particularly affecting the cervical spine, which is now affected as frequently as injuries to the thoraco-lumbar junction.

THE SKELETAL INJURY

In the *cervical spine* the injury most commonly complicated by damage to the spinal cord is a fracture–dislocation from a flexion–rotation force (see Fig. 8.1C). This usually occurs in the lower half of the cervical column, often between the fourth and fifth, or the fifth and sixth vertebrae. Dislocation of the atlanto-axial joint is occasionally responsible for cord damage, but this injury is usually fatal. In some cases of spinal cord injury in the neck there is no radiographic evidence of any bone injury or displacement: in such cases the nerve lesion may be caused by a protruded intervertebral disc (p. 105), by an infolded ligamentum flavum (p. 105), or possibly by momentary subluxation that has reduced spontaneously.

In the *thoracic and lumbar regions,* the skeletal injury responsible for damage to the spinal cord or cauda equina is nearly always a fracture–dislocation caused by a violent flexion or rotation force (Figs 9.3, 9.4 & 9.8).

Standard antero-posterior and lateral radiographs are required but seldom permit full assessment of the extent of the injury in either the neck or thoracic and lumbar regions. Computed tomography (CT scanning) provides excellent detail of the fracture pattern in the bone and will reveal the presence of any bony fragments within the spinal canal associated with cord compression (Fig. 10.1). When clinical examination reveals the presence of neurological injury, or where this is suspected, magnetic resonance imaging (MRI) is now the investigation of choice for evaluation of the spinal cord and associated soft tissues (Fig. 8.4B). It has now largely replaced contrast myelography for the evaluation of the extent of neurological damage and is available in all spinal injury centres.

THE NERVE INJURY

The character of the nerve lesion depends upon the site of the skeletal injury. In the *cervical region* the cord injury may be either complete or incomplete. Surprisingly, the extent of the nerve injury does not bear a constant relationship to the severity of the skeletal injury: severe cord damage may be found in the absence of any demonstrable bone injury and, conversely, there may be little or no neurological disturbance despite severe vertebral displacement. Neverthe-less, in most instances there is reasonable correlation between the degree of

Fig. 10.1 Computed tomographic (CT) scan in a case of burst fracture at the L1 level of the spine, showing marked encroachment by bone fragments on the spinal canal. There was a complete cauda equina lesion below the level of the fracture.

displacement and the severity of the nerve lesion. It is essential that a careful and complete neurological examination of motor and sensory function is performed on admission to provide a baseline record before any active treatment is undertaken.

In the *thoracic region* a fracture–dislocation usually causes complete transection of the spinal cord. Because of the anatomy of the facet joints and the stability provided by the rib cage, the force necessary to displace the vertebrae at this level is great. As a result, the spinal cord, which is soft and friable, is unable to withstand the shearing action of the displaced vertebra.

At the *thoraco-lumbar junction* (T12 to L1) the lowest segments of the spinal cord and the proximal roots of the cauda equina lie side by side in the spinal canal; so the nerve lesion caused by a fracture–dislocation may be a mixed one, due partly to cord injury and partly to nerve root injury (Fig. 10.2). If the lesion is incomplete it is nearly always the nerve roots rather than the cord whose function is preserved ('lumbar root escape').

In the *lumbar region* (below the first lumbar vertebra) the spinal cord has given place to the cauda equina, which is more resistant to injury than the spinal cord itself. In fracture–dislocations at this level the neural injury may therefore be incomplete.

Characteristics of complete transection of the cord. The immediate consequence of division of the cord is total suppression of function in the segments below the lesion (spinal shock). The initial paralysis is flaccid, there is complete sensory loss and the visceral reflexes are suppressed. This stage of spinal shock rarely lasts for more than 48 hours. As it gradually passes off, the paralysis becomes spastic instead of flaccid, and there is a return of exaggerated tendon and visceral reflexes unmodified by higher control. The end of this stage of spinal shock is signalled by the return of the bulbocavernosus reflex, which involves the S1, S2 and S3 nerve roots, is easily assessed and has important

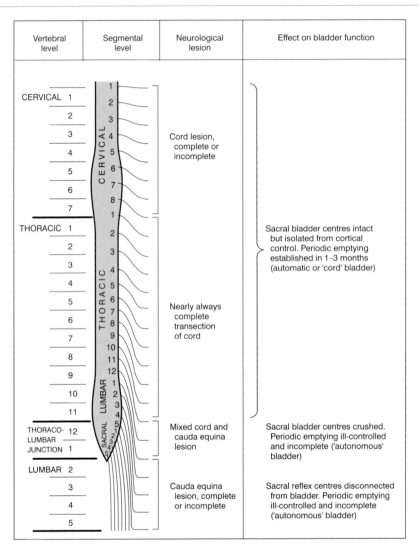

Vertebral level	Segmental level	Neurological lesion	Effect on bladder function
CERVICAL 1 2 3 4 5 6 7	CERVICAL 1 2 3 4 5 6 7 8	Cord lesion, complete or incomplete	
THORACIC 1 2 3 4 5 6 7 8 9 10 11	THORACIC 1 2 3 4 5 6 7 8 9 10 11 12 LUMBAR 1 2 3 4	Nearly always complete transection of cord	Sacral bladder centres intact but isolated from cortical control. Periodic emptying established in 1–3 months (automatic or 'cord' bladder)
THORACO- 12 LUMBAR JUNCTION 1	SACRAL 5 1 2 3 4 5	Mixed cord and cauda equina lesion	Sacral bladder centres crushed. Periodic emptying ill-controlled and incomplete ('autonomous' bladder)
LUMBAR 2 3 4 5		Cauda equina lesion, complete or incomplete	Sacral reflex centres disconnected from bladder. Periodic emptying ill-controlled and incomplete ('autonomous' bladder)

Fig. 10.2 Composite diagram showing the relationship between vertebral and segmental levels, the nature of the neurological lesion and the state of the bladder after vertebral injuries involving the spinal cord or cauda equina at various sites.

prognostic significance. The return of this reflex activity, without recovery of sensibility or voluntary motor power below the lesion, is diagnostic of complete transection of the spinal cord. Incomplete spinal cord lesions are indicated by the preservation of sacral sensation or reflexes in the S4 and S5 segments. Because of the temporary phenomena contributed by spinal shock, it is seldom possible to make an unequivocal diagnosis of complete transection of the cord until 48 hours or more after the injury, and accordingly repeated neurological examination is required in these first few days.

Characteristics of incomplete transection of the cord. The only certain sign of continuity of axons in the spinal cord is the preservation or early return of voluntary motor power and sensibility below the level of the lesion. Since the damage to the cord is predominantly anterior, special attention should be paid in examination to the detection of spared posterior column sensation or distal motor function.

Characteristics of severe injury to the cauda equina. The paralysis remains flaccid throughout. The tendon and visceral reflexes are abolished below the lesion and do not return unless the nerve fibres recover their function.

THE BLADDER

In the normal state, emptying of the bladder is governed by reflex centres in the second and third sacral segments of the spinal cord, with overriding control from the cerebral cortex. After transection of the cord above the sacral segments the overriding cerebral control is cut off, but the sacral reflex centres are left intact. In the early weeks after injury there is retention of urine, with overflow if the retention is not relieved. After an interval that varies from 1 to 3 months the reflex centres in the cord take over and control automatic emptying of the bladder when it is filled to a certain capacity. This reflex state has been termed automatic bladder or 'cord bladder'.

If the injury involves the sacral segments of the cord or the nerve roots that emerge from it in the cauda equine, the nerve pathways for reflex control of the bladder are severed. True reflex emptying does not occur. Instead, periodic emptying of the bladder is dependent upon a local reflex in the bladder wall itself. In this state of 'autonomous bladder' the emptying action of the detrusor muscle may have to be induced by manual compression of the abdominal wall or by abdominal straining, and the emptying is less complete than it is with an automatic or cord bladder.

SPECIAL DANGERS IN CASES OF SPINAL PARAPLEGIA

The main dangers in the early months arise from pressure sores developing in the ischaemic, insensitive skin, and from ascending infection of the urinary tract. Patients still die from these causes, especially if incorrectly managed, but with improved methods of treatment the mortality has been greatly reduced. The onset of spasticity can also lead quickly to the development of joint contractures, especially if facilities for skilled nursing and physiotherapy are not available.

PROGNOSIS

The spinal cord has no power of recovery after complete transection. On the other hand, after incomplete cord lesions a remarkable degree of recovery may sometimes occur despite severe initial paralysis. Recovery may continue for many months, but the earlier and the more rapidly it begins the better the prognosis. These incomplete lesions are more common in the cervical region than in the thoracic region, where complete transection is almost the rule.

The roots of the cauda equina behave like other peripheral nerves in their capacity for recovery: that is, they are able to recover or regenerate provided their sheaths remain patent and in continuity (see p. 63). Thus, if the injury is a *neurapraxia*, recovery may occur early. After *axonotmesis* the nerve fibres may regenerate, but the re-establishment of function depends upon their reaching healthy end-plates. *Neurotmesis* in this region is irrecoverable because surgical repair is hardly practicable.

It will be clear from what has been said that injuries of the cauda equina have a more favourable prognosis than cord injuries in three important respects: (1) the extent of the paralysis is less because the lesion is more distal; (2) the lesion is less likely to be a complete transection and (3) the chances of recovery of nerve function are much greater.

TREATMENT

In patients with acute spinal cord injury, improved neurological recovery has been reported when corticosteroids can be administered in high dosage in the first 8 hours following injury and continued for 24 hours. It is greatly to the patient's advantage if he or she can be admitted immediately to a special Spinal Injuries Unit, where the necessary facilities and staff for the management of these difficult cases are available. These are expensive resources and are therefore usually available only on a regional basis. Such centres are able to provide access to specialist advice from neurosurgeons, urologists, plastic surgeons and specialists in rehabilitation medicine, as well as orthopaedic surgeons. These facilities are combined with the availability of skilled nursing care and dedicated physiotherapy and occupational therapy.

Management of the fracture

In the case of *cervical injuries*, if bony displacement is present, reduction should be attempted by traction through skull calipers, as described on page 101. If CT scanning shows that displaced fragments of bone are encroaching upon the spinal canal (Fig. 8.4A), operative decompression may be required. When severe paralysis is present in the absence of bony displacement, MRI is required to eliminate protruded intervertebral disc material as a cause of spinal cord compression, because this may be amenable to operative excision.

In fracture–dislocation of the *thoracic spine* with total distal paralysis it is to be feared that the spinal cord is completely divided. Nevertheless, the surgeon cannot be certain that this is the case in the hours immediately after the injury, so there is an argument for operative correction of the displacement and internal fixation of the fragments, as described below. An increasing number of spinal injury centres now use early internal fixation of the unstable spine to facilitate earlier rehabilitation of the patient. The alternative, which is still acceptable but seldom used, is to disregard the fracture and to concentrate attention on skilful nursing, care of the bladder, and rehabilitation.

If the paralysis is incomplete, and particularly if it is increasing, appropriate scanning techniques are required to exclude any fragments of bone encroaching upon the spinal canal. If these are present, operative decompression by the antero-lateral or postero-lateral route, supplemented by internal fixation, is advisable.

In fractures lower down—that is, at the *thoraco-lumbar junction* or in the *lumbar region*—the neurological injury is more likely to be incomplete, at least some of the nerve roots being spared. When this is the case operation should be undertaken immediately. Its objects are: (1) to reduce any gross displacement under direct vision to ensure that the roots of the cauda equina are free from pressure or constriction and (2) to provide internal fixation of the fragments to prevent redisplacement and to facilitate nursing without a plaster. Internal fixation may be by Harrington rods, Luque rods, or pedicle screw fixation (Figs 9.6 & 9.7), as mentioned on page 114.

Nursing

A specialised nursing routine is essential if pressure sores are to be avoided. The old method of nursing the patient in a plaster bed has long been discarded, because it was found impossible to prevent the development of pressure sores in the anoxic and insensitive skin.

The accepted method now is to nurse the patient flat upon soft pillows. Every 2 hours throughout the day and night the patient is turned to a new position, to lie for equal periods upon the back and upon either side. Where available, a Stryker turning frame or electric bed should be used, because it reduces the demands on the nursing staff.

Gentle passive joint movements should be carried out regularly from an early stage to preserve mobility in the paralysed limbs and to prevent joint contractures. It is important, however, to avoid the use of force, which by damaging a joint may increase stiffness rather than overcome it (see p. 67), and may also promote the development of ectopic ossification in the paralysed muscles. Spasticity is sometimes a problem secondary to an upper motor neurone injury and may prove unresponsive to simple physiotherapy with a daily stretching routine. Pharmacological treatment with a presynaptic neurotransmitter inhibitor, such as baclofen, may be required in resistant cases.

Care and training of the bladder

In the first few days, during which a considerable volume of intravenous fluids may be required, the bladder may be drained by an indwelling Foley catheter in a closed system. After 1 or 2 weeks, when the fluid intake may be reduced, 4-hourly intermittent catheterisation should be substituted. No matter which method is used, great emphasis must be laid on the necessity for a strict aseptic technique when the catheter is changed. Some degree of bacterial colonisation is almost inevitable, but antibiotics should only be administered intermittently, when there is clear evidence of infection, with pyrexia, pyuria and an elevated leucocyte count.

Periodic emptying of the bladder should be encouraged from an early stage by allowing the bladder to fill almost to capacity between catheterisations and by draining it at regular intervals—usually four to six times a day.

In most cases of transection of the cord, satisfactory automatic emptying is established within 1–3 months of the injury. After irrecoverable damage to the sacral segments of the spinal cord or to the cauda equina, periodic spontaneous emptying is more difficult to establish and, because it is no longer governed by the reflex centres, the mechanism is less reliable. Micturition will have to be started or aided by abdominal straining or by manual compression, and a urinal may have to be worn permanently.

Rehabilitation

Despite severe permanent paralysis, the majority of patients with complete transection of the cord can be made reasonably independent and enabled to

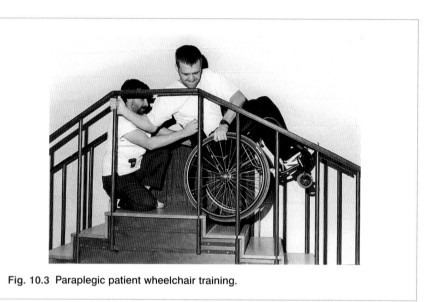

Fig. 10.3 Paraplegic patient wheelchair training.

Fig. 10.4 Paraplegic patient wheelchair training.

lead a useful life within the limits of their disability. Though some can walk short distances with calipers and crutches, for the most part they must get about permanently in wheelchairs. Early training should be undertaken to enable these patients to be confident and independent with the use of their wheelchairs in both indoor and outdoor conditions (Figs 10.3 & 10.4).

After cauda equina injuries, the possibilities of rehabilitation are much greater, especially when the nerve lesion is incomplete. Even when there is considerable irrecoverable damage, the patient can usually get about well with

Fig. 10.5 Ⓐ Bilateral full length leg orthoses to enable crutch walking. Ⓑ Spinal bracing in extension for trunk support.

elbow crutches or sticks, using appropriate lower limb orthoses (appliances) (Fig. 10.5A). Spinal bracing in extension may also be required to provide trunk support in the early stages of rehabilitation or following stabilisation of the thoraco-lumbar spine (Fig. 10.5B).

The advent of microchip computerised technology has opened up exciting new possibilities for assisted walking and standing in some younger para-plegic patients. The method, which is still experimental, uses functional elec-trical stimulation to produce cyclical contractions of the antigravity muscles which, with the assistance of orthotic bracing, can provide a limited form of reciprocal gait, or at least the ability to stand unaided.

Morale. An important part of the management of patients with traumatic paraplegic is the re-establishment of morale. It is natural that a person so afflicted may become seriously depressed and perhaps even feel that life can no longer be worth living. In such circumstances much depends upon the personality of the doctor with charge of the case, and upon the attitude of nursing and other paramedical staff. If the patient is fortunate enough to be in a centre established specially for the care of paraplegic patients, the fact of seeing other patients similarly afflicted, and especially of meeting those who are in the later stages of rehabilitation and who are already beginning to resume an active life, is always a considerable help to those recently injured. Later, the promotion of a competitive spirit among patients, with provision of

Fig. 10.6 Paraplegic patients engaged in wheelchair-aided group games.

facilities for games, has also proved to be a source of encouragement (Fig. 10.6). It is even more important to the patient, of course, if he or she can see some prospect of being able to get back to some form of remunerative employment, and facilities for retraining are normally part of the rehabilitation programme in such centres.

CLASSIFICATION

The injuries to be described may be classified as follows:

Fractures of the shoulder girdle

[1,2]	Fractures of the clavicle
[3]	Fractures of the body of the scapula
[4]	Fractures of the neck of the scapula
[5]	Fracture of the acromion process
[6]	Fracture of the coracoid process

Injuries of the shoulder and related joints
Dislocation of the sterno-clavicular joint
Strain of the sterno-clavicular joint
Subluxation and dislocation of the acromio-clavicular joint
Strain of the acromio-clavicular joint
Dislocation of the shoulder
Rupture of the tendinous rotator cuff of the shoulder

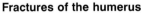

Fractures of the humerus

[1]	Fracture of the neck of the humerus
[2]	Fracture of the greater tuberosity
	Complex fractures of the upper end of the humerus
[3]	Fracture of the shaft
[4]	Supracondylar fracture
[5]	Fractures of the condyles
[6]	Fractures of the epicondyles

The most common injuries in this region are fracture of the clavicle, dislocation of the shoulder, fracture of the neck of the humerus and fracture of the shaft of the humerus. In children, fractures of the distal end of the humerus, at the elbow level, are common, and important because of the potential complications, which include damage to the brachial artery or median nerve and recalcitrant stiffness of the joint.

FRACTURES OF THE SHOULDER GIRDLE

The shoulder girdle comprises the clavicles and scapulae. Fractures of the clavicle are common and are caused by indirect violence. Fractures of the scapula are uncommon and are usually caused by direct violence.

FRACTURES OF THE CLAVICLE

Most fractures of the clavicle are caused by a fall onto the shoulder; occasionally a fall onto the outstretched hand is responsible. The most common site is at the junction of the middle and outermost thirds (Fig. 11.1). Less often a fracture occurs near the outer end of the clavicle. If displacement occurs—as it usually does—the lateral fragment is displaced downwards and medially in relation to the medial fragment (Fig. 11.1).

Treatment
The time-honoured method of holding the shoulders braced back by a figure-of-eight bandage has now been widely discarded. Its aim of bringing the fragments back into correct apposition is seldom realised, and it has the disadvantage that if the bandages are applied too firmly the venous return from the upper limb may be obstructed or—even more serious—one or more of the nerve trunks in the axilla may be constricted and injured. Most surgeons advise no more than support for the arm in a simple sling, for the relief of pain. The position of the fragments often remains imperfect, but moderate displacement does not hinder union and should be accepted. The sling should usually be worn for about 2 weeks (less in a child), but as soon as the initial

Fig. 11.1 Fracture of the clavicle at the usual site, with typical displacement.

sharp pain begins to subside—usually a week or so after the injury—active shoulder exercises should be begun, to restore full mobility.

Fractures of the clavicle unite readily, and the only common residual disability is a palpable or visible irregularity of the bone at the site of fracture. In children, remodelling quickly restores a normal contour. In adults some thickening may remain permanently, but it is seldom prominent. If the patient is seriously concerned about the cosmetic blemish, operative smoothing of bony prominences is justified. Operative reduction and internal fixation with an intramedullary pin or contoured plate is a practical alternative: the bony deformity is obviated but at the expense of a scar that may be prominent, so this operation is seldom advised. In the elderly there is a risk of stiffness of the shoulder if exercises are not practiced from an early stage.

The non-union rate following conservative management of fracture of the clavicle is less than 1%, but there may be an occasional indication for operative fixation to avoid this complication in widely displaced or severely comminuted fractures.

FRACTURES OF THE SCAPULA

The scapula is usually fractured by direct injury. Such fractures are uncommon and, in most cases, unimportant, because patients do well without special treatment. Nevertheless, these are often very painful injuries and there may be extensive extravasation of blood into the tissues, with widespread ecchymosis.

FRACTURE OF THE BODY OF THE SCAPULA

Although the fracture may be comminuted there is no important displacement because the fragments are held in position by their extensive muscle attachments both on the deep surface and on the superficial aspect of the bone.

Treatment. Attention should be directed mainly to the restoration of shoulder function. A sling is worn at first, but as soon as the pain begins to subside active shoulder exercises are begun, and continued until a full range of movement is regained.

FRACTURE OF THE NECK OF THE SCAPULA

The fracture extends from the scapular notch to the axillary border of the scapula, so that the part bearing the articular surface is detached in one piece from the body of the bone. The glenoid fragment may be displaced downwards, but displacement is seldom severe because the soft tissues help to retain the outer (glenoid) fragment in place.

Treatment. Again the main necessity is not to provide rigid splintage but to restore shoulder function by early active exercises as soon as pain allows. Indeed, immobilisation, except to the extent provided by a sling for the relief of pain, is unnecessary.

FRACTURE OF THE ACROMION PROCESS

The fracture occurs at a variable distance from the tip of the acromion. There may be no more than a crack without displacement, or the acromion may be comminuted and displaced downwards.

Treatment. If the fracture is simply a crack, or a comminuted fracture without displacement, it is sufficient to arrange active shoulder exercises as soon as the pain begins to subside; meanwhile a sling is worn.

If the acromion is badly comminuted, with much displacement of the fragments, operation to excise the acromion is advised. The proximal fringe of the deltoid muscle is reattached to the stump of the bone. After operation the arm is rested in a sling for 3 weeks and thereafter intensive mobilising exercises are begun.

Fracture of the coracoid process

The injury may be no more than a crack, or there may be a complete fracture with separation and downward displacement of the coracoid process.

Treatment. The fracture should be disregarded and attention concentrated on restoring shoulder function by early active exercises.

INJURIES OF THE SHOULDER AND RELATED JOINTS

DISLOCATION OF THE STERNO-CLAVICULAR JOINT

When the sterno-clavicular joint is dislocated the medial end of the clavicle is usually displaced forwards. The injury is uncommon. Rarely the clavicle is displaced backwards (retrosternal dislocation) and may press dangerously upon the trachea or great vessels.

Treatment. Anterior displacement is easily reduced by direct pressure over the medial end of the clavicle while the shoulders are arched forwards. A pad should be applied over the front of the joint and held in place by firm adhesive strapping. A sling is worn for 2 weeks, and thereafter active shoulder exercises are encouraged. The rare posterior dislocation demands early operative reduction: the displaced bone is pulled forward into place with a hook.

Recurrent dislocation

In a rather high proportion of cases, dislocation of the sterno-clavicular joint becomes recurrent or permanent despite early reduction of the first dislocation. In recurrent dislocation the clavicle springs forwards when the shoulders are braced back and clicks back into place when the shoulders are arched forwards.

Treatment. In most cases the disability is slight or negligible, and treatment is not required. In the occasional case in which the repeated displacement is troublesome, operation is advised. The joint may be stabilised by constructing a new retaining ligament from the tendon of the subclavius muscle or from a strip of fascia lata.

Strain of the sterno-clavicular joint

Strain of the sterno-clavicular joint is followed by local pain and swelling. The area of the joint is tender on palpation, but the clavicle is not displaced. Spontaneous recovery may be expected and no special treatment is required.

Strain of the acromio-clavicular joint

When the violence is insufficient to subluxate or dislocate the joint, a fall on the point of the shoulder may cause a strain of the joint capsule. There is pain localised accurately to the region of the joint, with marked tenderness on palpation. Pain is aggravated by attempted full abduction of the arm, which entails movement of the acromio-clavicular joint to the limit of its range.

Treatment. Recovery occurs spontaneously with time and use. A sling may be worn if pain is severe, but active shoulder exercises should be encouraged from the beginning.

SUBLUXATION AND DISLOCATION OF THE ACROMIO-CLAVICULAR JOINT

Injuries of the acromio-clavicular joint are much more common than injuries of the sterno-clavicular joint. A reason for this is that the joint, having a weak capsule, is inherently vulnerable in falls onto the shoulder. The joint depends for its integrity largely upon the accessory extra-articular (coraco-clavicular) ligaments, namely the conoid and trapezoid ligaments. Injuries are usually caused by falls onto the outer prominence of the shoulder, tending to force the acromion downwards. Such injuries are especially common among rugby football players.

Pathology

Subluxation. In cases of subluxation the capsule of the joint is torn and the acromion is displaced slightly downwards from the lateral end of the clavicle (Fig. 11.2A). Severe displacement is prevented by the intact conoid and trapezoid ligaments, which anchor the clavicle to the coracoid process.

Dislocation. When the joint is dislocated the mechanism is the same but the violence is more severe: the conoid and trapezoid ligaments are torn and the acromion is displaced markedly downwards (or the clavicle upwards) (Fig. 11.2B).

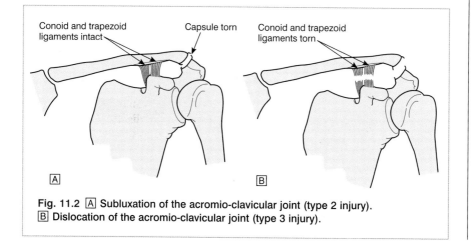

Conoid and trapezoid ligaments intact

Capsule torn

Conoid and trapezoid ligaments torn

A

B

Fig. 11.2 A Subluxation of the acromio-clavicular joint (type 2 injury). B Dislocation of the acromio-clavicular joint (type 3 injury).

Fig. 11.3 Stabilisation of the acromio-clavicular joint after dislocation. A screw is passed through a drill hole in the clavicle to engage the coracoid process.

Treatment

The time-honoured method in which encircling strapping is applied from the mid-part of the clavicle round the under side of the flexed elbow is not recommended: it is ineffective and unnecessary in cases of subluxation, and it is seldom adequate for a complete dislocation.

Subluxation. Disability from slight displacement of the acromio-clavicular joint is usually insignificant and may be accepted. The only treatment advised if pain is severe is to support the limb with a sling for 2 weeks or so, and to encourage active shoulder exercises from an early stage.

Dislocation. Because it is difficult to control a complete dislocation of this joint adequately by external splintage, operation should usually be advised. A simple method is to hold the clavicle in place by means of a screw passed through a drill hole in the clavicle to engage a pilot hole in the coracoid process (Fig. 11.3). Alternatively, reduction may be maintained by a stiff wire passed horizontally from the tip of the acromion, across the acromio-clavicular joint, into the clavicle. The screw or wire should be removed after 10 or 12 weeks, when it may be assumed that the torn ligaments will have healed.

Late reconstruction. In long-standing cases with high elevation of the outer end of the clavicle, reconstruction is advised. Among the best of current techniques is one in which the coraco-acromial ligament is detached from the acromion process and sutured to the stump of the clavicle after excision of its outer end (distal to the attachments of the conoid and trapezoid ligaments). After the operation, stability is ensured by means of a screw holding the clavicle to the coracoid process as described above.

DISLOCATION OF THE SHOULDER

The shoulder (gleno-humeral) joint is dislocated commonly in adults but seldom in children.

Pathology

For practical purposes dislocations of the shoulder may be grouped into two main types—anterior and posterior. Anterior dislocation is very much the more common. The cause is nearly always a fall onto the outstretched hand or onto

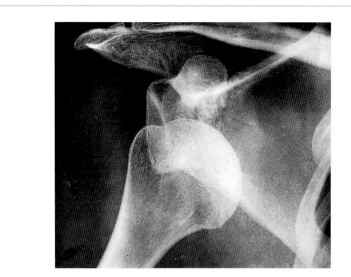

Fig. 11.4 Typical radiographic appearance in anterior dislocation of the shoulder.

the region of the shoulder itself. In most cases the humeral head is displaced through a rent in the capsule and comes to lie in the infraclavicular fossa just below the coracoid process: hence the term subcoracoid dislocation often used to describe this injury.

In the less common posterior dislocation there may be a history of a direct blow to the front of the shoulder, driving the humeral head backwards. More often, however, posterior dislocation is the consequence of an electric shock or an epileptiform convulsion, which perhaps acts by causing violent medial rotation. In such cases, both shoulders may be dislocated simultaneously.

Clinical features

Anterior dislocation. Pain is severe, and the patient is unwilling to attempt movements of the shoulder. On examination, the contour of the shoulder below the tip of the acromion—normally made strongly convex by the prominence of the humeral head—is flattened, so that the tip of the acromion is now the most lateral point of the shoulder region. A noticeable prominence, caused by the displaced humeral head, is seen and felt in the infraclavicular fossa. In very obese patients the characteristic features may be masked by the soft tissues, and unless care is taken, the dislocation may be missed on clinical examination: radiographic examination is always necessary. Radiographs show that the outline of the humeral articular surface is not congruous with the articular surface of the glenoid fossa (Fig. 11.4).

Posterior dislocation. The features of a posterior dislocation of the shoulder are not very striking, and for that reason the injury is often overlooked. An important sign is fixed medial rotation of the arm, which cannot be rotated outwards even as far as the neutral position. There is also flattening anteriorly below the front of the acromion, where the head of the humerus normally forms a

Fig. 11.5 A Antero-posterior radiograph in a case of posterior dislocation of the shoulder. Displacement is not obvious in this projection and might be overlooked, but note from the shape of its upper end that the humerus is rotated medially. This characteristic 'light bulb' appearance of the medially rotated bone is an important clue to the diagnosis. B The same shoulder after reduction of the dislocation, showing normal congruity of the joint surfaces.

rounded bulge. Radiography may be misleading if only the ordinary antero-posterior film is available, because the dislocation may not be apparent—or at least not obvious—in this projection (Fig. 11.5). It is, therefore, important, in doubtful injuries of the shoulder, to insist on a more detailed radiological study. A lateral projection, obtained by directing the rays upwards from the axilla, with the arm abducted to a right angle, is the most valuable, but if it is impossible to get the arm abducted widely enough for this examination, an oblique view will provide adequate visualisation of the gleno-humeral joint (Fig. 11.6).

Treatment

The dislocation should be reduced as soon as possible. An anaesthetic is usually necessary.

Anterior dislocation. The well-known Kocher[1] manoeuvre may still be used; the steps (slightly modified) are as follows: (1) with the elbow flexed to a right angle, steady but gentle traction is applied in the line of the humerus; (2) the arm is rotated laterally; (3) the arm is adducted by carrying the elbow across the body towards the midline; (4) the arm is rotated medially so that the hand falls across the opposite side of the chest.

[1] Theodor Kocher, a brilliant Swiss surgeon-anatomist, who was Professor of Surgery in Berne and was awarded the Nobel Prize in 1909. He described his technique for reduction of the dislocated shoulder based on cadaver studies in 1870.

Fig. 11.6 A Oblique view of a normal gleno-humeral joint taken with the tube angulated 30° from the vertical with the patient seated. B Oblique view using the same technique to diagnose posterior dislocation of the shoulder.

The alternative technique of reduction—now widely preferred—is to pull firmly and steadily upon the semi-abducted arm against counter-traction in the axilla, which may be provided either by an assistant or by the surgeon's stockinged foot; at the same time, direct backward pressure may be applied over the displaced humeral head by an assistant.

Reduction should be confirmed both by clinical tests and by radiographic examination. Thereafter the limb may be rested in a sling for a few days, but as soon as the pain has subsided active movements should be encouraged.

Posterior dislocation. Reduction is effected by rotating the arm laterally while applying longitudinal traction on the arm. Direct forward pressure may also be applied over the displaced humeral head. The after-treatment is the same as for anterior dislocation.

Complications

Injury to the axillary nerve. The axillary (circumflex) nerve is often damaged in anterior dislocations of the shoulder, with a reported incidence of 5–30%. There is consequent paralysis of the deltoid muscle, with a small area of anaesthesia at the lateral aspect of the upper arm. It is important that axillary nerve function be checked and the result recorded before any attempt at reduction of the dislocation. Treatment is expectant, as for other nerve injuries complicating closed injuries of the limbs (p. 63). Recovery in a few weeks or months is the rule, but if the nerve has been severely damaged by traction the changes may be irreversible and the paralysis permanent.

Other nerve injuries. Occasionally other branches of the brachial plexus are damaged, especially the posterior cord.

Vascular injury. In anterior dislocation the displaced humeral head may occasionally damage the axillary artery, especially if the vessel is atheromatous; or the artery may be damaged during attempted late reduction of a dislocation that has been overlooked.

Associated fracture. Dislocation of the shoulder is often accompanied by fracture of the greater tuberosity of the humerus. Treatment is not difficult, because once the dislocation has been reduced the fracture may be treated along the usual lines.

A more serious association is that between dislocation of the shoulder and fracture of the neck of the humerus. Again the plan of treatment should be first to reduce the dislocation (if necessary by operation) and then to deal with the fracture.

Recurrent anterior dislocation of the shoulder

In some instances the damage sustained by a shoulder in a violent dislocation is permanent and of such a nature that it predisposes to further dislocations. These tend to occur with increasing frequency and with decreasing violence. Recurrent instability is far more common in younger patients under the age of 40 who experience their first dislocation as the result of a sporting injury. Too early mobilisation and return to sporting activity may also predispose to redislocation.

Pathology
Whereas in ordinary or non-recurrent dislocation of the shoulder there is probably a tear of the capsule which heals spontaneously when the dislocation has been reduced, in recurrent dislocation the pathology is different, and is such that spontaneous healing does not occur (Figs 11.7 & 11.8). The changes are twofold: (1) the inferior labrum and capsule are stripped from the anterior margin of the glenoid rim forming the Bankart[2] lesion and (2) the articular surface of the humeral head is dented postero-laterally (probably from violent impingement against the sharp anterior margin of the glenoid fossa) (Figs 11.7 & 11.8).

Recurrent dislocation occurs most easily when the arm is abducted, extended and rotated laterally, allowing the defect in the articular surface of the head to slip over the front of the glenoid.

Diagnosis
This is largely based on the history. Radiographic demonstration of a humeral head defect is confirmatory evidence. In a doubtful case the precise nature of

---

[2] Blundell Bankart, a technically brilliant English orthopaedic surgeon working in London, described the shoulder lesion in recurrent dislocation and the operation for its repair in 1923.

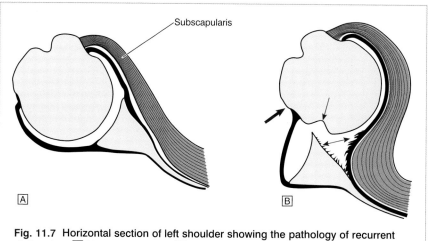

Fig. 11.7 Horizontal section of left shoulder showing the pathology of recurrent dislocation. A Normal condition. B The humeral head is shown dislocated forwards. It has stripped the capsule from the anterior margin of the glenoid, creating a pocket in front of the neck of the scapula into which the humeral head is displaced. Note that the humeral head has been dented (arrow) by the sharp glenoid margin. The defect thus caused in the articular surface is a typical feature.

Fig. 11.8 A Typical defect of the articular surface of the humeral head (arrow), found in most cases of recurrent dislocation of the shoulder. B Radiographic appearance. The defect is seen at the upper and outer quadrant of the humeral head as a vertical edge of compacted bone (arrow). It is shown best when the arm is in medial rotation, as in this radiograph.

Fig. 11.9 CT scan of shoulder after the injection of contrast, showing a large anterior pocket where the capsule and periosteum have been stripped from the bone. Note also the small fragment detached from the anterior margin of the glenoid fossa.

the pathology may be demonstrated by computed tomographic (CT) scanning after the injection of contrast medium into the joint (Fig. 11.9), or by arthroscopy.

Treatment

If the disability is troublesome, operation is advised. Many operations have been advocated, but the two most commonly used both depend upon a repair of the deficient anterior tissues. In the Putti-Platt[3] operation the subscapularis muscle is shortened by overlapping or 'reefing' to limit lateral rotation. In an alternative operation, that of Bankart, the detached capsule and glenoid labrum are reattached to the front of the glenoid rim. Arthroscopic techniques have been developed, allowing closed repair of the labrum and capsule with suture anchors, and are likely to be used increasingly in the future.

RUPTURE OF THE TENDINOUS (ROTATOR) CUFF OF THE SHOULDER

(Torn supraspinatus)

As age advances, the tendinous cuff of the shoulder, of which the supraspinatus tendon forms the central part, degenerates and is liable to rupture if subjected to sudden stress, as from a fall onto the shoulder or even from an everyday action such as pushing a heavy door. The tendinous cuff includes the supraspinatus tendon and the adjoining flat tendons that are blended with it, namely the infraspinatus behind and the subscapularis in front. They form a cuff over the shoulder that has also been termed the rotator cuff. Distally, the tendons forming the cuff blend with the capsule of the shoulder.

A clear distinction must be made between major tears of the tendinous cuff and minor tears or strains.

---

[3] Vittorio Putti, Professor of Orthopaedics in Bologna, and Sir Harry Platt of Manchester, later President of the Royal College of Surgeons of England, were jointly credited with developing this operation in 1923.

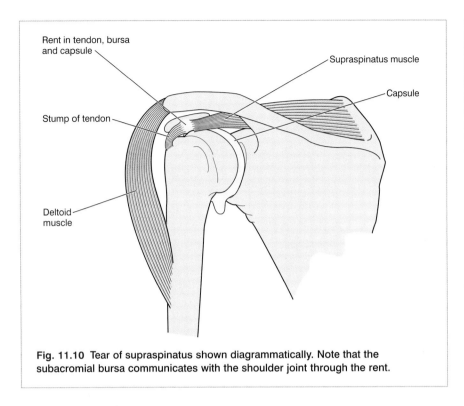

Rent in tendon, bursa
and capsule

Supraspinatus muscle

Capsule

Stump of tendon

Deltoid
muscle

Fig. 11.10 Tear of supraspinatus shown diagrammatically. Note that the
subacromial bursa communicates with the shoulder joint through the rent.

Major tears

After a major tear of the cuff (Fig. 11.10) the action of the supraspinatus muscle
is lost. The clinical features are characteristic. The patient is unable to initiate
abduction of the shoulder because the early phase of abduction demands the
combined action of the supraspinatus (which stabilises the humeral head in
the glenoid fossa) and the deltoid (which lifts the arm); but when the arm is
raised passively to the right angle the patient can sustain abduction by deltoid
action alone (Fig. 11.11).

Treatment. When the patient is elderly, as is often the case, operation should
usually be avoided, because the degenerate nature of the tendon makes satisfactory repair impracticable. Even though untreated, some patients eventually
regain the ability to abduct the arm by deltoid action alone. In younger patients
operative repair is advised. It entails exposure of the tendon from above by
splitting the acromion in the coronal plane, and repair or reattachment of the
tendon by sutures through holes drilled in the tuberosity of the humerus.
Thereafter a long course of supervised exercises may be required before a full
range of active movement is restored. As would be expected, the results of
operation tend to be poorer in cases of large musculo-tendinous defects than
when the rent is small. Synthetic materials are now becoming available to patch
large defects and arthroscopic techniques are under development for the closed
repair of smaller tears.

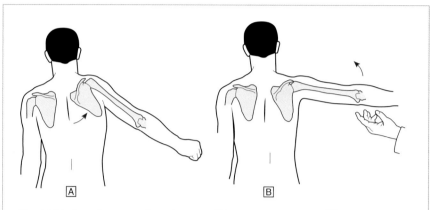

Fig. 11.11 Complete tear of tendinous cuff (torn supraspinatus). [A] Active abduction from the resting position is possible only by rotation of the scapula; there is no active abduction at the gleno-humeral joint, because the deltoid is unable to initiate abduction without the help of the supraspinatus. [B] When the limb is raised passively beyond the horizontal, abduction can be sustained actively by the deltoid muscle.

Minor tears

If the tendon is only strained, the action of the supraspinatus is not lost. There is a full range of active shoulder movement, but there is pain during the mid-part of the range of abduction, caused by impingement of the damaged part of the tendon beneath the acromion process or coraco-acromial ligament. A minor tear of the supraspinatus is thus one cause of the well-known 'painful arc' syndrome (supraspinatus syndrome); for a full description, the reader is referred to textbooks on orthopaedics. Treatment is conservative, by rest, short-wave diathermy and graduated exercises.

FRACTURES OF THE HUMERUS

FRACTURE OF THE NECK OF THE HUMERUS

Fracture of the neck of the humerus occurs most often in elderly women, in whom it is a common injury. In a high proportion of such persons there is some degree of rarefaction of the skeleton from osteoporosis, so that the bones are relatively weak. This type of fragility fracture is usually caused by a fall onto the limb. Displacement is variable: there may be none, or there may be moderate or severe tilting of the head fragment so that the shaft appears either abducted or adducted in relation to it (Fig. 11.12A). A notable and favourable feature is that in well over half the cases the fragments are firmly impacted together so that the bone moves as one piece. Impaction is important because it has a bearing on treatment.

Diagnosis

The fracture may easily be overlooked if it is impacted, because the patient may be able to use the arm to some extent without severe pain. The possibility of a fracture should always be suspected from the nature of the injury—especially

Fig. 11.12 Ⓐ Fracture of the neck of the humerus with moderate displacement. Radiographs do not indicate with certainty whether such a fracture is impacted or not, but this is easily decided by clinical examination (see text). Ⓑ Extensive bruising gravitating down the arm, a feature typical of these fractures.

when the patient is an elderly woman—and after a day or two from the appearance of extensive bruising in the upper and middle parts of the upper arm (Fig. 11.12B). (The visible bruise tends to gravitate down the arm, and may extend almost to the elbow after a few days.)

Radiographs do not indicate with certainty whether or not the fracture is impacted. This can best be determined by clinical examination. If the limb can be handled and moved passively through a reasonable range without causing severe pain, the fracture is impacted, whereas if the slightest attempt to move the limb causes severe pain the fracture is not impacted.

Treatment

In a discussion on the best method of treatment of this injury three points should be borne constantly in mind: first, that even severe displacement is compatible with the restoration of function that is fully adequate for an elderly person; secondly, that it is often impossible to hold the fragments in normal relationship except by an extensive plaster or by operation; and thirdly, that the shoulder is prone to become stiff if it is immobilised for a long time, especially in elderly persons. In most cases, therefore, the most satisfactory method of treatment is that which permits early mobilisation of the shoulder, even if this means that an imperfect position of the fragments must be accepted. As with all other fragility fractures, it is important that once the injury has been treated, the patient should be investigated to detect and treat any severe underlying osteoporosis as outlined in Chapter 6.

Standard conservative method. In the usually elderly victim of this injury, displacement should be ignored and attention concentrated on the restoration of function. Whether or not immobilisation is necessary will depend upon the state of the fracture.

Impacted fractures. If the fracture is impacted, immobilisation is unnecessary. Active and assisted shoulder movements should be begun immediately and continued daily, the arm being carried in a sling in the intervals between treatment.

Unimpacted fractures. If the fracture is not impacted, immediate shoulder exercises are impracticable because of the pain that movement causes. The arm should be supported in a sling, supplemented by a body bandage to hold the arm to the chest wall for the first week. Elbow, wrist and finger exercises should be practised from the beginning, but shoulder movements are deferred for 2 or 3 weeks, when the sling may be worn outside the clothes. By that time the fragments are generally glued together sufficiently by granulation tissue to allow assisted shoulder exercises with little or no pain, and without fear of retarding union.

Alternative surgical methods for special cases. Although a result adequate for an elderly patient can be achieved when even considerable displacement is left unreduced, in younger patients there is a place for deliberate reduction if the fragments are in poor position. Reduction can often be achieved by manipulation under anaesthesia, the distal (shaft) fragment being brought into line with the head fragment. To maintain reduction it is sometimes necessary to immobilise the limb on an abduction frame for 4 weeks.

Operative reduction is required in less than 15% of fractures when it is impossible to secure a satisfactory reduction by manipulation, especially when the neck fracture is associated with a fracture of the greater tuberosity ('three-part fracture') (Fig. 11.13A) or with dislocation of the shoulder. If operation is resorted to, internal fixation should be used to secure the fragments. The choice lies between a metal plate fixed with screws (Fig. 11.13B), or tension band wiring. In either case it may be difficult to secure rigid fixation because of the small size of the proximal fragment. In a more severely comminuted three- or four-part fracture, where there is a significant risk of avascular necrosis or non-union, there may be a place for immediate replacement arthroplasty by the substitution of a metal humeral prosthesis for the damaged natural head (Fig. 11.14).

Complications

Joint stiffness. In elderly persons the shoulder is prone to become stiff after injuries in the vicinity of the joint, especially if it is immobilised for a long time. Hence, it is important to get the shoulder moving by active or assisted exercises as soon as the condition of the fracture will allow. The sooner movements can be begun the less is the risk of serious stiffness.

Arterial injury. There is a serious risk of impalement of the brachial artery upon a sharp fragment of bone, especially when the shoulder is dislocated. This may cause an acute vascular emergency, or it may lead to traumatic aneurysm with progressive vascular and neurological insufficiency.

Fig. 11.13 Ⓐ Severe fracture of the neck of the humerus in an adult of middle age. The greater tuberosity is also detached. Ⓑ After open reduction and fixation of the fragments with a plate and screws.

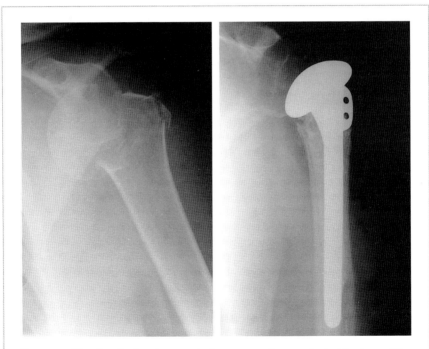

Fig. 11.14 Neer hemiarthroplasty replacing a severely comminuted fracture of the humeral head with a metal-stemmed prosthesis.

Nerve injury. Occasionally a fracture of the neck of the humerus is complicated by injury to the axillary nerve, evidenced by the patient's inability to contract the deltoid muscle during attempted abduction of the shoulder, and by numbness or anaesthesia over a small area at the outer side of the upper arm.

Treatment is expectant (p. 63). Gradual recovery is usually observed.

Exceptionally, there may be damage to the brachial plexus, either from direct impact on the nerves when the shoulder is dislocated, or from progressive stretching of nerves over a traumatic aneurysm of the brachial artery.

Dislocation of the shoulder. Rarely the fracture is associated with dislocation of the shoulder.

Treatment. The dislocation should be reduced first (if necessary by operation) and the fracture should then be treated along the usual lines.

FRACTURE OF THE GREATER TUBEROSITY OF THE HUMERUS

Fracture of the greater tuberosity is usually caused by a fall onto the shoulder. It occurs in adults of any age, but particularly in the elderly. Usually there is no marked displacement (Fig. 11.15), but the tuberosity may be comminuted. In a few cases a fragment of bone is lifted away from the tuberosity by the action of the attached muscles and is separated widely from its bed.

Treatment

The treatment depends on whether or not the tuberosity fragment is severely displaced. If it is not—as is usually the case—splintage is unnecessary and all

Fig. 11.15 Fracture of the greater tuberosity of the humerus. In this case there was no displacement of the fragment. Sometimes the fragment is avulsed from its bed and pulled upwards by the muscles attached to it.

that is needed is to arrange shoulder exercises to restore movement and function.

If a fragment of bone is avulsed and separated widely from its bed in the tuberosity, the problem of treatment is more difficult. Accurate reduction of the displacement is essential if full function of the shoulder is to be restored. It may be possible to replace the separated fragment in position by abducting the arm, but it is difficult to maintain the position without holding the limb abducted in a cumbersome plaster or splint. It is, therefore, usually advisable to undertake operative reduction and internal fixation by a screw. In the convalescent period shoulder exercises should be practised until satisfactory function is restored.

Complications

Painful arc syndrome (supraspinatus syndrome). Thickening or irregularity of the greater tuberosity may interfere with free abduction at the gleno-humeral joint, because the thickened area may impinge against the acromion process or coraco-acrominal ligament, with consequent pain. Impingement occurs mainly during the middle phase of abduction.

Treatment. In most cases the symptoms gradually subside under prolonged treatment by exercises. Exceptionally, if severe symptoms persist, there is a place for excision of the acromion.

FRACTURE OF THE SHAFT OF THE HUMERUS

The shaft of the humerus is usually fractured in its middle third, either from an indirect twisting force (which causes a spiral fracture) or from direct violence (which causes a transverse, short oblique, or comminuted fracture). The fracture occurs in adults of any age, but seldom in children. Displacement is variable: there may be no loss of position, or there may be marked angulation or overlapping of the fragments (Fig. 11.16A&B).

The proximal half of the humerus is a common site for pathological fracture from carcinomatous metastases.

Treatment

Provided the alignment of the fragments is good, it is unnecessary to secure perfect end-to-end apposition. Contact over one-third or one-half of the area of the fracture is sufficient. Nor is it usually necessary to enforce strict immobilisation, because most of these fractures unite readily with a minimum of external splintage.

Standard method. If displacement is greater than can be accepted, reduction is carried out by manipulation under anaesthesia. A plaster is applied to maintain alignment of the fragments, but as a rule it need not give absolute immobility. Most surgeons rely upon a plaster cylinder encircling only the upper arm from the axilla to the elbow (Fig. 11.17A). Further support can be provided by a sling. Alternatively, a prefabricated brace, held in place by Velcro straps, which compresses the soft tissues and permits unlimited motion of the shoulder and elbow joints, may be applied (Fig. 11.17B). Assisted shoulder exercises and active finger exercises should be practised under the supervision of a physiotherapist.

Once the fracture is becoming 'sticky'—indicating that union is occurring—a well-moulded cast-brace of plastic material or plaster that allows mobility of the elbow as well as of the shoulder may be all that is required.

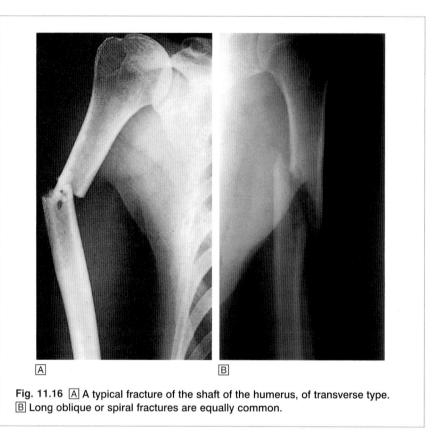

Fig. 11.16 A A typical fracture of the shaft of the humerus, of transverse type. B Long oblique or spiral fractures are equally common.

Alternative methods for special cases. When the fragments are very unstable, or in the case of a pathological fracture from a metastatic tumour, a more positive method of fixation is required. Internal fixation may be effected by a plate and screws applied to the shaft or—often better when the fracture is near the middle of the shaft—by an intramedullary nail, preferably combined with locking screws. The nail is preferably inserted from below, entering just above the olecranon fossa: insertion from above, through the greater tuberosity, may impair shoulder movement. It is usually possible for the nailing to be done 'closed' using intra-operative radiographic screening. It is rarely necessary to expose the fracture itself, unless there is associated nerve or arterial injury or significant interposition of soft tissue.

In the case of a contaminated open fracture, or of an infected fracture, preference should be given to external fixation by means of twin threaded pins inserted percutaneously into each fragment, the pins then being held rigidly to an external metal bar by clamps (see p. 42).

Complications

Nerve injury. Injury to the radial nerve is frequent because of its close contact with the bone as it winds round its posterior aspect, and occurs in 10–15% of

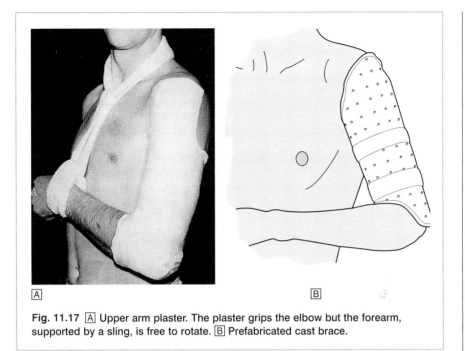

Fig. 11.17 Ⓐ Upper arm plaster. The plaster grips the elbow but the forearm, supported by a sling, is free to rotate. Ⓑ Prefabricated cast brace.

fractures of the shaft of the humerus. The nerve injury is usually no more than a contusion, seldom complete division. The effects of paralysis of the radial nerve in the upper arm are chiefly motor: there is paralysis of the extensor muscles of the wrist, fingers and thumb ('wrist-drop'), and of the brachio-radialis and supinator. The only sensory change is a small area of anaesthesia or blunting of sensibility on the radial side of the back of the hand.

Treatment. The principles of treatment of nerve injuries complicating fractures were considered in Chapter 4 (p. 63). In closed fractures it is assumed that the nerve is in continuity and spontaneous recovery is awaited. If reinnervation of the most proximal muscle has not occurred in the expected time, as calculated from the distance from the site of injury to the neuromuscular junction, the nerve should be explored. In most cases of injury to the radial nerve the prognosis is good. In neglected cases, or when repair of a divided nerve is impracticable, adequate function may be restored by suitable tendon transfers. A satisfactory plan is as follows: the pronator teres is transferred to the extensor carpi radialis brevis to extend the wrist; flexor carpi ulnaris or flexor carpi radialis is transferred to the extensor digitorum and extensor pollicis longus to extend the fingers and thumb; and palmaris longus is transferred to the abductor pollicis longus to provide abduction of the thumb away from the palm.

Non-union. Although most fractures of the shaft of the humerus unite readily despite imperfect immobilisation, there are a few that are extremely obstinate and defy the ordinary methods of conservative treatment, no matter for how long they are continued. Indeed, the mid-shaft of the humerus is recognised as a site of some of the most recalcitrant cases of non-union (Fig. 11.18).

Fig. 11.18 Non-union of a nailed fracture of the humerus A before and B after treatment by plating and grafting.

Treatment. If it is clear that union is not occurring with conservative treatment a bone-grafting operation, with or without internal fixation, should be advised. Cancellous onlay grafts may be combined with fixation by a long intra-medullary nail or by a plate and screws. In a particularly obstinate case there is a place for treatment by electrical stimulation.

SUPRACONDYLAR FRACTURE OF THE HUMERUS

Supracondylar fracture of the humerus is one of the most common and important fractures of childhood. It is seldom seen in adults. It should always be regarded as potentially dangerous because of the risk of injury to the brachial artery.

The injury occurs through a fall onto the outstretched arm. Displacement, when it occurs, is characteristic: the lower fragment is displaced backwards and tilted backwards (Fig. 11.19).

Treatment

Undisplaced fractures in children require no more than 3 weeks' protection in plaster. When the fragments are displaced, manipulative reduction under anaesthesia should be undertaken (Fig. 11.20). The lower fragment is brought back into position by longitudinal traction on the limb and direct pressure behind the olecranon with the elbow flexed 90° or more. Perfect anatomical reposition is not essential provided any lateral tilting of the lower fragment is corrected, because remodelling can gradually efface a moderate displacement as the bone grows. After reduction the limb is immobilised in plaster with the elbow flexed a little more acutely than the right angle.

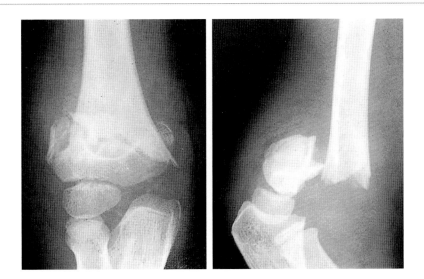

Fig. 11.19 Supracondylar fracture of the humerus in a child, showing the typical displacement.

Fig. 11.20 The same elbow as in Fig. 11.19, after manipulative reduction of the displacement.

When the fracture is unstable, internal fixation by two percutaneous pins is recommended. The first wire enters through the lateral condyle and passes obliquely upwards and medially to engage the medial humeral cortex. The medial wire enters through the medial epicondyle and is passed obliquely upwards and laterally: the two wires cross just above the olecranon fossa.

Precautions

A careful watch should be kept on the condition of the circulation in the forearm and hand. The plaster should be cut away at the radial side of the wrist to allow the surgeon to feel for the radial pulse.

Complications

The main importance of this fracture lies in the risk of damage to the brachial artery, a possibility that must always be borne in mind. Other complications include injury to the median nerve, and mal-union with consequent deformity.

Arterial occlusion. Injury to the brachial artery by the sharp upper fragment may lead to impairment of the circulation to the forearm and hand (Fig. 11.21). The artery may be severed or simply contused. If it is contused, its lumen may be occluded by thrombosis or, rarely, by spasm of the vessel wall.

The effects of arterial occlusion at the elbow vary from case to case. In a small proportion the circulation is impaired so severely that gangrene of the digits ensues. More often, enough blood gets through the collateral vessels to keep the hand alive, but the flexor muscles of the forearm, and sometimes the peripheral nerve trunks, may suffer ischaemic changes. The affected muscles are gradually replaced by fibrous tissue, which contracts and draws the wrist and fingers into flexion (Volkmann's[4] ischaemic contracture) (Fig. 11.22). If the peripheral nerve trunks are also damaged by ischaemia, there will be sensory and motor paralysis in the forearm and hand, which may be temporary or permanent according to the severity of the ischaemic damage.

Diagnosis. In the incipient stage vascular occlusion is suggested by signs of impaired circulation in the hand and fingers (see p. 21), and particularly by the patient's inability to extend the fingers fully, with marked pain in the forearm

Fig. 11.21 Shows how a supracondylar fracture of the humerus may damage the brachial artery, with risk of consequent ischaemia in the forearm and hand. The artery is shown obstructed at and below the point of impact. Ischaemia may also be caused by overtight plaster or dressings.

[4] Richard von Volkmann was a German surgeon with an international reputation who was Professor in Halle, Saxony and also served as an Army surgeon in the Franco-Prussian War. He described the process of ischaemic muscle paralysis and contracture in 1881.

Fig. 11.22
Typical
appearance of
the hand in
established
Volkmann's
ischaemic
contracture.

Shoulder and upper arm

if passive extension is attempted. This is a most important test that should always be carried out. A positive finding should immediately arouse suspicion of arterial damage. In the established stage the diagnosis is clear from the history and the characteristic flexion contracture of wrist and fingers (Fig. 11.22).

Treatment. In the incipient stage the problem is that of dealing with a sudden occlusion of the brachial artery. The case must be handled as an emergency, because the effects of the occlusion become irreversible after a few hours. The following action must be taken:

- First step. Any external splint or bandage that might be causing constriction is removed. Displacement of the fragments, if not already reduced, is corrected so far as possible by gentle manipulation. Heat cradles or hot bottles are applied over the other three limbs and trunk to promote general vasodilation. If these measures fail to bring about a return of adequate circulation within half an hour, the next step is taken.
- Second step. At operation the brachial artery is explored. If the occlusion is due to kinking or spasm of the artery, an attempt is made to relieve it by freeing the vessel and applying papaverine. If this fails, the artery may be distended by the injection of saline between clamps. As a last resort, the artery may have to be opened and damaged intima removed, repair being effected thereafter with a vein patch; or a bridging vein graft may be required. Any operative intervention for this serious complication should include decompression of the anterior fascial compartment of the forearm (see Compartment syndrome, p. 63). Whenever possible, such operations should be carried out only by surgeons with experience of vascular surgical techniques.

In the established stage restoration to normal is impossible because important muscles have been irretrievably damaged: reconstructive surgery at best can only improve what function remains. The choice of treatment depends upon the circumstances of each case. In mild cases, acceptable function may be restored by intensive exercises guided by a physiotherapist, but such cases are uncommon. In the usual more severe cases the muscle shortening may be counteracted by detachment and distal displacement of the flexor muscle origin (muscle slide operation). In selected cases with severe muscle infarction, however, the best results are probably obtained by excision of the dead muscles and subsequent transfer of a healthy muscle (for example, a wrist flexor or extensor) to the tendons of flexor digitorum profundus and flexor pollicis longus to restore active flexion of the digits. These muscle transfers may be combined, in appropriate cases, with arthrodesis of the wrist. When the median nerve is irreparably damaged by ischaemia, nerve grafting is sometimes successful in restoring its function.

Injury to the median nerve. The median nerve is occasionally injured by the protruding lower end of the proximal fragment, just as the brachial artery may be damaged. Treatment should be expectant at first, on the assumption that the lesion is no more than a neuropraxia (p. 63).

Deformity from mal-union. It has been mentioned already that in children it is not essential to restore perfect anatomical apposition of the fragments, because remodelling will gradually efface a moderate backward or lateral shift of the lower fragment. However, an alteration of alignment cannot be corrected spontaneously, so if a fracture has been allowed to unite with appreciable tilting of the distal fragment there will be permanent deformity. The most common deformity to be seen clinically is outward bowing at the site of fracture, causing cubitus varus (Fig. 11.23A).

Treatment. When the deformity is slight it can usually be accepted, but if the angulation is marked it should be corrected by osteotomy in the supracondylar region of the humerus (Fig. 11.23B).

Fig. 11.23 Ⓐ Cubitus varus after a supracondylar fracture of the humerus in which medial tilting of the lower fragment was left uncorrected. Ⓑ Radiograph after corrective osteotomy.

CONDYLAR FRACTURES IN THE ADULT

Isolated supracondylar fractures are less common in adults than children, but are usually caused by much greater violence. This may be a fall on the point of the elbow or from direct trauma in motor vehicle collisions when the driver has rested his elbow through an open window. As a result, the fracture has a more complex T- or Y-shaped configuration (Fig. 11.24) with involvement of one or both condyles and occasionally dislocation of the elbow joint.

Treatment

In the occasional simple transverse supracondylar fracture conservative treatment may be possible by closed manipulation and immobilisation in a plaster cast with a flexed elbow. However, the majority of adult fractures extend into the articular surface of the elbow joint demanding open reduction and internal fixation to allow early restoration of movement. These operations are technically demanding and should only be undertaken by those who are familiar with the necessary surgical approach and the use of the appropriate contoured plates and screws to achieve stabilisation. In the elderly patient the osteoporotic bone may lack the strength to allow the use of these implants without risk of early loosening. The only alternative is to use multiple Kirschner wire fixation supported by external splintage for 3–6 weeks and to accept a less perfect position and a stiff joint.

Complications

Stiffness. The elbow joint is notorious for the rapid development of postoperative stiffness and this can only be avoided by early mobilisation, preferably with a continuous passive motion machine.

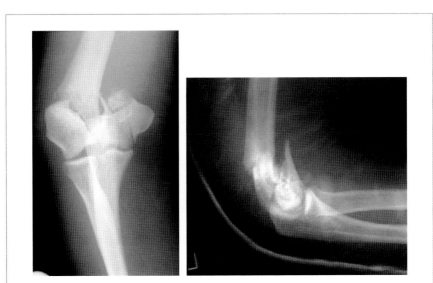

Fig. 11.24 Comminuted supracondylar fracture showing Y-shaped configuration.

Osteoarthritis. The development of secondary osteoarthritis is common and is often accompanied by disabling pain. In severe cases the only long-term solution may be to undertake joint arthroplasty.

Arterial injury. As with the childhood fracture, the brachial artery is at risk of injury from sharp bony fragments at the fracture site.

FRACTURES OF THE CONDYLES OF THE HUMERUS

Condylar fractures are relatively uncommon, but often troublesome. Like supracondylar fractures, they occur mainly in children. The usual cause is a fall. The lateral condyle is fractured much more commonly than the medial, and the description that follows relates mainly to injuries of the lateral condyle.

The usual lateral condylar fracture (fractured capitulum) extends obliquely upwards and laterally from the capitular surface. In young children the greater part of the detached fragment may be cartilaginous, so that the fragment appears much smaller as seen radiographically than it is in fact (Fig. 11.25). Displacement is seldom severe, but even moderate displacement is important because the fracture involves the joint surface.

Treatment

A simple crack fracture without displacement requires no more than protection for a few weeks in plaster, followed by a course of mobilising exercises for the elbow.

Fig. 11.25 Fracture of the lateral condyle of the humerus. In children (the usual victims of this injury) the lower end of the humerus is largely cartilaginous and therefore invisible on radiographs. What might appear on the radiographs to be a minor flake fracture in fact represents the injury shown in the diagram, with separation of a large fragment including the whole of the articular surface of the capitulum. Accurate reduction is essential.

Displaced fractures must be regarded seriously because they are potentially a cause of permanent disability. An attempt should be made first to reduce the displacement by manipulation under anaesthesia. If this is successful a plaster is applied with the elbow at 90° and retained until union occurs.

If manipulation fails to give perfect reduction, operation is advised. The fracture is exposed and reduced under direct vision, and the condylar fragment is fixed in position by a small screw (a Herbert dual-pitch scaphoid screw may be appropriate) driven from the lateral aspect of the detached fragment obliquely into the expanded lower end of the humerus.

Complications

Condylar fractures are prone to non-union, and may lead to deformity of the elbow and to osteoarthritis.

Non-union. The fracture line remains clearly visible and the condylar fragment—usually consisting of a large part of the capitulum—is displaced slightly upwards (Fig. 11.26).

Treatment. If non-union is recognised before the elbow has become seriously disorganised by persistent displacement of the condylar fragment, operation is advised. The fracture surfaces are freshened and brought accurately into position, and the condylar fragment is secured with autogenous bone pegs or a screw. In neglected cases with long-established non-union, the disability may have to be accepted. The elbow is already considerably disorganised and function is unlikely to be improved by late operation.

Deformity. Deformity at the elbow may be caused by persistent upward displacement of the fractured condyle, or by retardation of epiphysial growth on the affected side from damage to the growing epiphysial cartilage. If the lateral condyle is affected the deformity will be that of cubitus valgus, whereas involvement of the medial condyle causes cubitus varus.

Fig. 11.26 Fracture of the lateral condyle of the humerus with persistent non-union 8 years after the injury. The separated condyle (capitulum) is displaced slightly upwards.

Treatment. If the deformity is slight it may be accepted, but if angulation is marked it should be corrected by supracondylar osteotomy of the humerus (Fig. 11.23B).

Frictional neuritis of the ulnar nerve. In cases of cubitus valgus there is a risk of ulnar paralysis from frictional neuritis where the nerve is angled behind the medial epicondyle. If symptoms of ulnar neuritis develop, the nerve should be transposed from its post-epicondylar groove to a new bed in front of the elbow.

Osteoarthritis. Osteoarthritis is liable to occur when a condylar fracture leaves permanent deformity or irregularity of the articular surface. As a rule it does not become troublesome until several years after the original injury, and if the elbow is not subjected to heavy stress the arthritis may never cause serious disablement.

FRACTURES OF THE EPICONDYLES

Whereas most condylar fractures affect the lateral side, epicondylar fractures usually affect the medial (Fig. 11.27). The injury occurs rather more often in children than in adults. It may be caused by direct violence, but it is often an avulsion injury, the epicondyle being pulled off by the attached flexor muscles during a fall; this latter type is usually associated with dislocation or momentary subluxation of the elbow.

Treatment

In an uncomplicated case only symptomatic treatment is required. Displacement is seldom severe and need not be corrected. The elbow should be immobilised in plaster for 3 weeks to relieve pain, and thereafter joint movement should be restored by active exercises. In the occasional case in which the fragment is widely displaced, operation may be advisable: it is sufficient to hold the fragment back in place by sutures through the adjacent soft tissues.

Fig. 11.27 Fracture of the medial epicondyle of the humerus. There was transient damage to the ulnar nerve.

Complications

The important complications are: (1) inclusion of the medial epicondylar fragment in the elbow joint and (2) injury to the ulnar nerve.

Inclusion of epicondylar fragment in the joint. This complication occurs in children. The separated fragment of the medial epicondyle is 'sucked' into the joint cavity and may become jammed between the joint surfaces (Fig. 11.28). The fragment is not completely loose and free within the joint: it retains its attachment to the forearm flexor muscles.

Treatment. It is imperative that the fragment be removed from the joint. Sometimes, with the patient anaesthetised, it may be extracted by extending fully the wrist and fingers to put the flexor muscles on the stretch, while the joint is widened at the medial side by abduction of the forearm and the negative pressure within the joint is released by the insertion of a hollow needle. Open operation is thus avoided. If this manoeuvre fails, operation is required. After the fragment has been extracted by operation it should be secured in the normal position by sutures through the overlying soft tissues.

Injury to the ulnar nerve. The ulnar nerve is clearly in danger of immediate direct injury in displaced fractures of the medial epicondyle. It may also suffer gradual damage later, from friction upon a roughened groove.

Treatment. Whenever there is interference with the ulnar nerve at the elbow it should be transposed from its groove behind the medial epicondyle to a new bed in the soft tissues at the front of the elbow.

Fig. 11.28 Avulsion of the medial epicondyle with inclusion of the fragment in the joint. Operation was required to release the fragment.

12 | Elbow and forearm

CLASSIFICATION

Injuries of the elbow
    Dislocation of the elbow
    Dislocation of the head of the radius
    Subluxation of the head of the radius
    Contusion of the elbow

Fractures of the forearm bones

[1] Fracture of the olecranon process
[2] Fracture of the coronoid process
[3] Fracture of the head of the radius
[4] Fracture of the upper end of the ulna with dislocation of the head of the radius (Monteggia fracture-dislocation)
[5] Fracture of the shafts of the forearm bones
    Fracture of the shaft of the radius with dislocation of the inferior radio-ulnar joint (Galeazzi fracture-dislocation)
[6] Fracture of the lower end of the radius
    Fracture of the lower end of the radius with anterior displacement
    Fracture-separation of the lower radial epiphysis

Injuries of the elbow and forearm are common in both adults and children. They may be caused by direct violence to the arm, as in a road accident or assault, or by indirect violence from a fall onto the hand. The injuries will be classified by their anatomical site, though it should be noted that damage to the elbow joint and forearm fractures may sometimes occur together.

INJURIES OF THE ELBOW

DISLOCATION OF THE ELBOW

Dislocation of the elbow is usually caused by a heavy fall onto the outstretched hand. It is a fairly common injury both in children and in adults.

Pathology

The dislocation is nearly always posterior or postero-lateral (Fig. 12.1). That is to say, the ulna and the radius are displaced backwards, or backwards and laterally, relative to the humerus. There may be an associated fracture of the coronoid process of the ulna, or of the radial head, capitulum or medial epicondyle, but in most such cases the fracture is of a minor nature.

Treatment

The dislocation should be reduced under anaesthesia as soon as possible. Reduction is usually easy: all that is necessary is to pull steadily upon the forearm with the elbow semi-flexed, while direct pressure is applied behind the olecranon. Reduction should be confirmed by radiographic examination and clinical tests: the radiographs should be scrutinised for one or more of the fractures mentioned above. Thereafter it is recommended that the elbow be rested in a plaster backslab in 90° of flexion for 2 weeks before mobilising

Fig. 12.1 Postero-lateral dislocation of the elbow in an adult.

exercises are begun. A plaster affords the best conditions for healing of the injury to the soft tissues, which is often extensive; furthermore, it allows greater freedom of movement at the shoulder and hand than does the collar-and-cuff sling that is often prescribed for this injury.

Complications

Vascular or nerve injury. Occasionally the brachial artery or one of the major nerve trunks is damaged in a dislocation of the elbow, but when the severity of the displacement is considered it is remarkable how uncommon these complications are. The treatment of injuries to the brachial artery was considered on page 62, and the treatment of closed nerve injuries on page 64.

Joint stiffness. The elbow is prone to troublesome stiffness after injury, and especially after dislocation. The stiffness is usually caused by intra-articular and peri-articular adhesions (p. 65), and it will gradually yield to active exercises, provided they are persevered with for long enough. Manipulation and passive stretching should be avoided: the elbow never lends itself well to manipulation and, indeed, stiffness may often be made worse thereby.

A less common but more serious cause of stiffness is post-traumatic ossification (wrongly termed myositis ossificans), a condition in which new bone forms in the haematoma beneath the stripped-up periosteum and joint capsule (Fig. 12.2). The treatment of this complication was considered on page 67.

Fig. 12.2 Ossified haematoma (so-called myositis ossificans) about the elbow after a fracture–dislocation.

DISLOCATION OF THE HEAD OF THE RADIUS

Very occasionally the head of the radius may be dislocated forwards without any disturbance of the humero-ulnar relationship and without a fracture. The injury is probably caused by forced pronation. Reduction should be attempted by supinating the forearm while direct pressure is applied over the displaced radial head.

Caution. It should be noted that dislocation of the head of the radius as an isolated injury is rare, and that it is more often associated with a fracture of the shaft of the ulna (Monteggia fracture, p. 171). Radiographic examination should always include the whole length of the ulna lest a fracture be overlooked.

The head of the radius is sometimes congenitally dislocated, in which case it tends to be somewhat globular and lacks the normal concavity of its upper articular surface. Care must be taken to avoid confusing this congenital deformity with a traumatic dislocation. It is useful to know that a congenital dislocation, which is rare, is likely to affect both elbows similarly.

SUBLUXATION OF THE HEAD OF THE RADIUS (Pulled elbow)

If a young child is lifted by the wrist the head of the radius may be pulled partly out of the annular ligament. This injury is sometimes termed 'pulled elbow'. There is local pain, and movements of the elbow are restricted. The displacement is easily reduced by pushing the forearm upwards and rotating it alternately into supination and pronation.

CONTUSION OR STRAIN OF THE ELBOW

In children an injury of the elbow may cause severe pain and limitation of movement even in the absence of bone injury or displacement. The lesion is probably a strain of the capsule or a contusion of the articular cartilage or periosteum. The only treatment required is rest for 2 weeks in a plaster or sling, followed by active exercises. As in all elbow injuries, manipulation and passive stretching should be avoided.

FRACTURES OF THE FOREARM BONES

FRACTURE OF THE OLECRANON PROCESS

The olecranon is fractured by a fall onto the point of the elbow, usually in an adult. The fracture may take three forms (Fig. 12.3): a crack without displacement; a clean break with separation of the two fragments; or a comminuted fracture. The fracture line nearly always enters the joint near the middle of the trochlear notch.

Treatment

The treatment depends upon the type of fracture, and will be considered in relation to the three types mentioned above.

Crack fracture. The only treatment necessary is to protect the elbow by a light plaster splint for 2 or 3 weeks. It is unnecessary to apply the plaster with the

Elbow and forearm

Fig. 12.3 Fractures of the olecranon and their treatment. The diagrams in the upper row show the three types of fracture, and those below depict the treatment for each type. A Crack without displacement. Treatment—rest in plaster. B Clean break with separation. Treatment—open reduction and fixation by screw or by a tension band wire. C Comminuted fracture. Treatment—excision of fragments and re-attachment of triceps.

elbow fully extended; the joint may safely be flexed to a right angle without fear of distracting the fragments, which are held together by the surrounding aponeurosis. The right-angled position is more comfortable for the patient and it allows functional activity of the hand and fingers.

Clean fracture with separation. It is impracticable to gain and hold perfect reduction by closed methods because the action of the triceps will angulate and distract the fragments, so operation should be advised. The fragments are exposed and fitted together accurately under direct vision, with care to ensure that the articular surface of the trochlear notch is perfectly smooth. Rigid fixation is attained by a long, coarse-threaded cancellous screw passed down the bone from the upper surface of the olecranon (Fig. 12.3B), or by short stiff parallel wires driven vertically across the fracture, combined with a tensed figure-of-eight loop of wire ('tension band wiring') (Figs 12.3B & 12.4). The wiring technique has the advantage of maintaining better fixation by increasing axial compression of the fracture during elbow flexion. Depending upon the degree of stability obtained, it may or may not be advisable to protect the elbow in plaster for 2 weeks before mobilising exercises are begun.

Comminuted fracture. Perfect replacement and fixation of the fragments are usually impracticable, though it is sometimes possible to achieve acceptable

Fig. 12.4 $\boxed{\text{A}}$ Displaced fracture of the olecranon. $\boxed{\text{B}}$ The olecranon fracture after open reduction and fixation by a tension band wire, with restoration of the articular surfaces.

fixation by the use of a contoured plate and screws. The more frequent treatment for this type is to excise the olecranon fragments by dissecting them out from the aponeurosis that forms the insertion of the triceps, and to secure the triceps to the stump of the ulna by strong sutures passed through small drill holes in the bone (Fig. 12.3C). After operation the elbow is protected in plaster for 3 weeks and thereafter mobilised by active exercises.

Complications
These are: (1) non-union, (2) mal-union and (3) osteoarthritis.

Non-union. Olecranon fractures usually fail to unite by bone if a gap is allowed to remain between the fragments. The gap is bridged by fibrous tissue, so the continuity of the triceps is restored. Nevertheless, the power of extension is weakened. In elderly patients the disability can usually be accepted. In younger persons it may be advisable to excise the scar tissue, freshen the fracture surfaces, and secure the fragments in close apposition by a long screw.

Mal-union. For practical purposes the fracture is described as mal-united if the fragments unite in such a way that there is a 'step' or irregularity in the articular surface of the trochlear notch. Its significance lies in the fact that it may predispose to the later development of degenerative arthritis (osteoarthritis). If the deformity of the articular surface is only slight, the situation is usually best accepted. Only if there is severe deformity in a young person would operation be considered. Operation would entail either osteotomy, repositioning of the misplaced fragment and fixation by a cancellous screw, or excision of the proximal fragment, if it is small.

Osteoarthritis. Osteoarthritis may develop some years after the injury if the articular surface of the olecranon is left roughened or 'stepped'. The arthritis is unlikely to become severe enough to produce significant pain and elbow stiffness unless the arm is used for heavy work.

FRACTURE OF THE CORONOID PROCESS

The coronoid process is seldom fractured except in association with posterior dislocation of the elbow. Marked displacement is prevented by the strong aponeurotic fibres, prolonged from the insertion of the brachialis muscle, that invest the bone. No special treatment is needed other than that for the associated dislocation.

FRACTURE OF THE HEAD OF THE RADIUS

Fracture of the head of the radius is one of the most common fractures of the upper limb in young adults. It is caused by a fall onto the outstretched hand in pronation, the force being transmitted axially along the shaft of the radius with impaction of the radial head against the capitulum. In most cases the fracture is no more than a vertical crack without displacement (Fig. 12.5): in most of the remainder, a segment of the disc-shaped radial head is broken away and

Fig. 12.5 Fracture of the head of the radius without displacement. Note the vertical crack extending downwards from the articular surface. Rest in plaster is the only treatment required. In these minor injuries the fracture line is often ill-defined and may easily be overlooked.

Fig. 12.6 A Fracture of the head of the radius with comminution. B After excision of head of radius. Comminution severe enough to justify operation is uncommon.

depressed below the plane of the articular surface. Sometimes the whole of the head is extensively comminuted (Fig. 12.6A). The cartilage covering the articular surface is often badly bruised, as is also the articular cartilage of the capitulum, a feature that is not evident from the radiographs.

Diagnosis

A fracture of the head of the radius is easily overlooked because it is sometimes not immediately obvious in the radiographs, particularly when the fragments are impacted. Features that should suggest the true nature of the injury are a history of a fall onto the outstretched arm, with marked local tenderness on palpation over the head of the radius, and restriction of elbow movement, especially of forearm rotation, with sharp pain at the lateral side of the joint at the extremes of rotation. If in the presence of these symptoms and signs a fracture is not seen on the initial radiographs, further films should be obtained to show the radial head in different positions of rotation. It is also essential to examine the wrist to exclude damage to the distal radio-ulnar joint.

Treatment

The treatment required depends upon the severity of the damage to the radial head. In most cases the damage is slight rather than severe.

Slight damage. If radiographs suggest that the radial head has been only slightly damaged with minimal separation of the fragments, and that after union has occurred the articular surface will be reasonably smooth, conservative treatment is recommended (Fig. 12.5). A light plaster is applied with the elbow at a right angle and with the forearm midway between pronation and supination. The plaster is worn for 2–3 weeks until the pain settles, after which active mobilising exercises are arranged. A plaster is preferred to the more usual collar-and-cuff sling, because it eliminates pain and allows freer use of the shoulder and hand.

Severe damage. If the radial head is severely comminuted, with inevitable permanent distortion of the articular surface, operation should be advised (Fig. 12.6). If internal fixation of the fragments with small screws is impractical, the entire head of the radius should be excised. When the fracture is associated with a dislocation of the elbow excision should be deferred for 3 months to reduce the risk of the development of ectopic ossification (myositis ossificans). After operation the elbow is rested in plaster for 2 weeks before active mobilising exercises are begun. In selected cases of displaced fracture without gross comminution in active individuals, there has been a recent trend towards operative reduction and internal fixation, in order to prevent possible proximal migration of the radius. Fixation is achieved either with a miniature plate screwed to the lateral aspect of the neck, or by a Herbert dual-pitch headless screw.

Replacement of the radial head by a metal or non-metallic prosthesis as an alternative to simple excision is still on trial, and its place in management is not yet established.

Fractures in children. In children the fracture is usually through the neck of the radius, often with tilting of the radial head. Reduction is achieved by manipulation or, if necessary, by operation. Excision of the radial head should never be advised in children, because as growth occurs the radius is liable to ride up towards the humerus, with consequent disturbance of its relationship to the ulna.

Complications

Complications are infrequent: usually the function of the elbow is restored to normal or almost so. Occasional complications are: (1) joint stiffness and (2) osteoarthritis.

Joint stiffness. The range of flexion-extension and of rotation movement at the elbow may be impaired for a long time after a badly comminuted fracture even when it has been treated promptly by excision of the radial head. In most cases the stiffness yields slowly but surely to active exercises if they are carried out with sufficient perseverance. It should be remembered that the elbow is a joint that does not tolerate manipulation or forced passive movements. Indeed, recovery may be retarded rather than hastened by the injudicious use of force in an attempt to increase the range, especially in children.

Osteoarthritis. If the articular surface of the radial head is left roughened and irregular, wear and tear of the joint will be accelerated and osteoarthritis may supervene. It is partly to forestall this complication that excision of the radial head is recommended in cases of severely comminuted fracture. In the early stage, when arthritis is incipient rather than established, timely excision of the radial head may delay its progress. When osteoarthritis is established, excision of the radial head cannot be expected to bring full relief.

Fig. 12.7 The Monteggia fracture–dislocation, a combination of fracture of the upper half of the ulna with dislocation of the head of the radius. The displacement is usually forwards, as shown here, but the reverse deformity may occur.

FRACTURE OF THE UPPER END OF THE ULNA WITH DISLOCATION OF THE HEAD OF THE RADIUS (Monteggia[1] fracture–dislocation)

This uncommon injury is usually caused by a fall associated with forced pronation of the forearm, but a similar injury may be caused by a direct blow on the back of the upper forearm, as in a person warding off an assault. The usual displacement is characteristic: the distal ulna is angled forwards and the head of the radius is dislocated forwards (Fig. 12.7). Rarely, the reverse deformity occurs.

Treatment

For this complex injury, accurate reduction is essential and is seldom possible using closed methods, except occasionally in children. The radial head can usually be reduced into the annular ligament by full supination, but operation is normally required to reduce and fix the ulna fracture with a plate and screws. The elbow and forearm should then be immobilised in a plaster cast at a right angle for 4–6 weeks. In the rare event where the postoperative radiograph shows incomplete reduction, an open reduction may be necessary.

---

[1] Giovanni Monteggia was Professor of Surgery in Milan and described the fracture-dislocation of the forearm in 1814 before the advent of radiology.

FRACTURES OF THE SHAFTS OF THE FOREARM BONES

A fracture may involve either the radius alone or the ulna alone, or both bones. These injuries will be considered together because similar principles of treatment apply to them all.

The cause may be either an indirect force such as a fall onto the hand, or a direct blow on the forearm. Displacement may be absent or slight, but these fractures are notoriously prone to severe displacement, which is often very difficult to correct without open operation (Fig. 12.8). In general, displacement is more frequent and more severe in adults than in children, who often sustain no more than a greenstick fracture with minor angulation.

Treatment

In fractures of the forearm bones, accurate reduction is important because even slight residual displacement may disturb the relationship between radius and ulna, with consequent impairment of rotation, and often with subluxation of the inferior radio-ulnar joint.

Fig. 12.8 A A typical fracture of both bones of the forearm, with marked displacement. B After manipulative reduction and immobilisation in plaster. Though successful in this case, manipulation often fails to restore an acceptable position, and operative reduction will then be required.

Fig. 12.9 Full-length arm plaster with elbow flexed 90°. This is the standard type of plaster for many injuries of the elbow and forearm.

Conservative treatment. In children, and sometimes also in adults, it is worthwhile first to attempt manipulative reduction under anaesthesia. If this is successful a full-length arm plaster is applied with the elbow at a right angle and the forearm in a position midway between pronation and supination (Fig. 12.9). Check radiographs should be taken weekly for the first 3 weeks to ensure that redisplacement within the plaster does not go undetected. The plaster is retained until union occurs, usually a matter of 10 or 12 weeks in an adult.

Operative treatment. In a high proportion of cases, especially in adults, it is impossible to obtain satisfactory reduction by manipulation, or to maintain reduction by splintage in plaster. Failure is almost inevitable when the plane of the fractures is oblique or spiral. In these cases, operative reduction and internal fixation are required.

The fracture is exposed and the fragments are fitted together accurately under direct vision. If both the radius and the ulna are injured they should be approached through separate incisions. Internal fixation is effected usually by a metal plate held by six screws, three in each fragment (Fig. 12.10). The alternative use of an intramedullary nail to fix the ulna fracture is not recommended in adults, as the control of axial alignment is less satisfactory than with a plate. It can sometimes be used in children where rigid fixation is less essential and introduction through the olecranon process results in less soft tissue damage at the fracture site. Whether or not the additional protection of a plaster is required depends upon the rigidity of the fixation that has been achieved. If stability is in doubt it is wise to have the safeguard of a full-length arm plaster (Fig. 12.9), especially for the first few weeks.

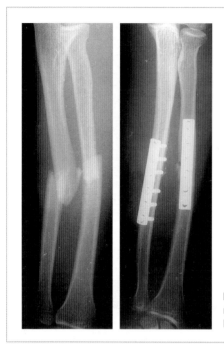

Fig. 12.10 Fractures of the shafts of the radius and ulna before and after fixation by plates and screws.

Complications

As with any bone that lies superficially beneath the skin, there is a risk of infection from contamination of an open fracture. Another possibility that must always be borne in mind is vascular occlusion from soft-tissue swelling within a rigid plaster or within a fascial compartment (Compartment syndrome, p. 63). These emergencies require very prompt treatment if the function of the limb is to be preserved. Complications that are seen more often are delayed union, non-union and mal-union.

Delayed union and non-union. Fractures of the shafts of the forearm bones are prone to delayed union or non-union (Fig. 12.11A), and this applies particularly to the ulna near the junction of its middle and lowest thirds. In most cases the cause is believed to be either impairment of the blood supply to one of the fragments, or imperfect immobilisation with consequent rotatory shearing movement between the fragments.

Treatment. Most cases of delayed union or non-union of the forearm bones lend themselves well to bone-grafting operations. If the fragments remain in good position and alignment it may be sufficient to lay slivers of cancellous bone from the ilium under the periosteum without disturbing the fracture itself (Phemister graft; see p. 56). If the position of the fragments is imperfect the fracture surfaces should be cleared of fibrous tissue, full reduction should be obtained under direct vision, and the fracture should be rigidly immobilised with a plate and screws. At the same time iliac cancellous bone grafts should be laid around the fracture to stimulate bone healing. When neither bone is

Fig. 12.11 Treatment with plate and graft for non-union of the radius and delayed union of the ulna. A Fracture of radius not united 10 months after injury and plating. B Sound consolidation of the radial fracture after replating and bone grafting.

united they should each be grafted at the same operation through separate incisions to avoid the risk of cross union. After operation a plaster may or may not be required, depending upon the rigidity of the fixation.

Mal-union. It has been emphasised already that without operation it is often difficult or impossible to secure accurate coaptation of the fragments in fractures of the forearm bones. If an imperfect position is accepted there is a risk of impaired function of the forearm and wrist, particularly in rotation, and the more severe the mal-position the more likely it is to cause trouble.

Impairment of function may arise in three ways: it may be caused by angulation of the fragments, by relative shortening of one of the bones, or occasionally by cross union between the radius and ulna. Angulation of the radius or ulna, or of both bones, can produce a mechanical block to rotation beyond a certain limited range. Cross-union between the two bones, of course, prevents rotation altogether. Shortening of one of the two bones, or unequal shortening of both bones, leads to subluxation at the inferior radio-ulnar joint, with consequent pain and restriction of movement.

Treatment. In many cases slight or moderate disability from mal-union can be accepted. Only occasionally is it justifiable to reproduce the fracture at operation in order to restore correct apposition and alignment. Pain and stiffness from subluxation of the inferior radio-ulnar joint may be relieved by excising the lower end of the ulna (see Fig. 12.22).

FRACTURE OF THE SHAFT OF THE RADIUS WITH DISLOCATION OF THE INFERIOR RADIO-ULNAR JOINT
(Galeazzi[2] fracture–dislocation)

In this injury the shaft of the radius is fractured near the junction of its middle and lowest thirds, the ligaments of the inferior radio-ulnar joint are ruptured and the head of the ulna is displaced from the ulnar notch of the radius. The fragments of the radius are usually tilted medially towards the ulna (Fig. 12.12). The head of the ulna may be shifted medially, anteriorly or posteriorly. The injury is analogous to the Monteggia fracture–dislocation in the upper part of the forearm (p. 171): it is said to be more common than the Monteggia injury. The cause is usually a fall onto the hand.

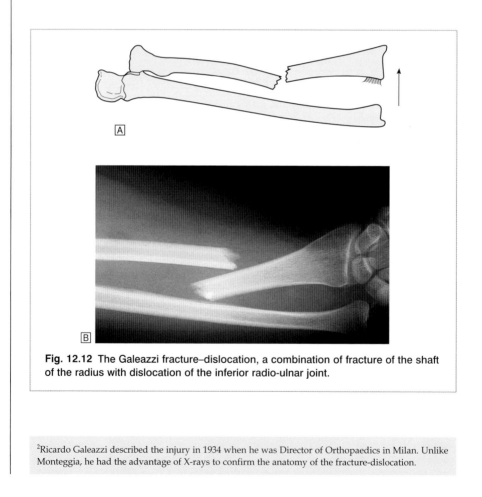

Fig. 12.12 The Galeazzi fracture–dislocation, a combination of fracture of the shaft of the radius with dislocation of the inferior radio-ulnar joint.

[2]Ricardo Galeazzi described the injury in 1934 when he was Director of Orthopaedics in Milan. Unlike Monteggia, he had the advantage of X-rays to confirm the anatomy of the fracture-dislocation.

Treatment

Perfect reduction is essential for restoration of full function. Only occasionally —and then usually in children—can adequate reduction be gained and maintained by conservative methods. In adults redisplacement is common after reduction by manual traction and supination, so resort must usually be had to operative reduction and internal fixation of the radial fracture, preferably by a metal plate with screws. Once the radius has been secured in anatomical position, stable reduction of the inferior radio-ulnar dislocation is usually achieved without difficulty. The position is held by a full-length arm plaster with the elbow flexed to the right angle and the forearm supinated: the plaster is retained until union occurs.

FRACTURE OF THE LOWER END OF THE RADIUS (Colles's fracture)

The Colles's[3] fracture is seen more often than any other injury in fracture clinics in civilian practice. It is not the most common fracture at all ages–indeed, it occurs rather infrequently in young adults–but it is certainly the most common fracture in persons over 40 years of age, and especially in women. The association of the fracture with osteoporosis is now well established and it is frequently the first indication of the presence of a generalised loss of bone mass. The condition and its association with the other so-called 'fragility fractures', particularly those of the vertebral bodies and proximal femur, is described more fully in Chapter 6 (p. 79). The fracture is nearly always caused by a fall onto the outstretched hand.

The typical deformity

In a few cases there is simply a crack without displacement, but in the great majority the fracture and displacement are characteristic. The fracture occurs transversely about 2 cm above the lower articular surface of the radius. The lower fragment is displaced slightly backwards and laterally and is tilted backwards, so that the articular surface, instead of pointing downwards and slightly forwards as in the normal wrist, is directed downwards and backwards (Figs 12.13–12.16). The lower fragment is also driven upwards and impacted into the upper fragment. Sometimes a vertical extension from the main transverse fracture enters the articular surface of the wrist joint. The styloid process of the ulna is commonly detached, but not always.

This typical displacement is reflected in a characteristic clinical appearance that has been termed the 'dinner-fork' deformity (Fig. 12.14). There is a dorsal hollow or depression in the lowest third of the forearm (proximal to the fracture), but immediately below this there is a marked prominence caused by the lower fragment's being displaced backwards, carrying with it the whole of the carpus and hand. Anteriorly there is fullness where the soft tissues are stretched over the forward-projecting upper fragment.

---

[3]Abraham Colles, a Dublin surgeon, published a report on Fracture of the Carpal Extremity of the Radius in 1814. It should be remembered that at that time X-rays were not available, and it is probable that the injury, though often seen, had previously been confused with dislocation of the wrist.

Fig. 12.13 The typical displacement in Colles's fracture. The distal fragment of the radius is tilted backwards so that the articular surface is directed downwards and backwards instead of downwards and slightly forwards as in the normal state. The distal fragment is often also shifted backwards, as depicted here. The normal state is shown for comparison, with the level of the fracture indicated by interrupted line.

Fig. 12.14 Typical 'dinner-fork' deformity from displaced fracture of the lower end of the radius (Colles's fracture).

Reversed deformity

In a small proportion of fractures of the lower end of the radius the deformity is the reverse of that described above. That is, the lower fragment is displaced forwards and rotated forwards so that the articular surface is directed too far anteriorly. This variation, known as Smith's fracture, is described separately on page 187.

Treatment

In displaced fractures the standard method of treatment is to undertake manipulative reduction under either local or general anaesthesia and to immobilise the forearm and wrist in a below-elbow plaster. In effecting the reduction the fragments must first be disimpacted and the bone drawn out to full length; the distal fragment can then be repositioned accurately by firm pressure over its dorsal surface (see Fig. 12.18).

Technique of reduction. The muscles of the forearm should be relaxed, either by general anaesthesia (supplemented if necessary by a relaxant) or by regional anaesthesia. The first step is to disimpact the fragments, which have often been driven together firmly in the position of deformity. Disimpaction is achieved by

Fig. 12.15 A typical Colles fracture of the lower end of the radius. Note in the lateral view the backward displacement and backward tilt of the lower fragment, whose articular surface now points downwards and backwards. In this case the styloid process of the ulna is intact: commonly it is fractured near its base.

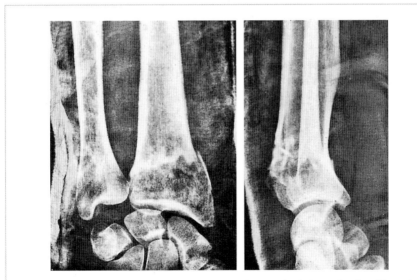

Fig. 12.16 The fracture seen through plaster after manipulative reduction. Normal alignment is restored. Note in the lateral radiograph that the articular surface of the radius is directed downwards and slightly forwards-the normal orientation.

Fig. 12.17 First step in the reduction of a fracture of the lower end of the radius with backward tilting of the distal fragment: traction is being applied to disimpact the fragments.

Fig. 12.18 The 'thenar grip' recommended for correcting the backward displacement and tilting of the distal fragment of the radius. Note the position of the surgeon's hands: the thenar eminence of one hand is placed over the distal fragment to press it forwards against the counter-pressure of the other thenar eminence upon the shaft of the radius just above the fracture. It will be found easiest to use the right hand to control the distal fragment when the fracture involves the left radius (as shown here), and the left hand in a fracture of the right radius.

firm longitudinal traction upon the hand and thumb, against the counter-traction of an assistant who grips the arm above the flexed elbow (Fig. 12.17). When the fragments have been disimpacted, their mobility can be demonstrated by grasping the distal fragment between the finger and thumb of one hand and the proximal fragment likewise with the other hand. Reposition of the distal fragment may then be achieved by firm forward pressure (best applied by the thenar eminence) over the distal fragment, with counter-pressure (directed backwards) against the proximal fragment just above the fracture. This key manoeuvre is illustrated in Figure 12.18. After reduction a plaster is applied with the wrist in the neutral position between

Fig. 12.19 Dorsal plaster slab, a usual method of immobilisation for a fracture of the lower end of the radius. The slab covers the dorsum and sides of the forearm and wrist. It is secured firmly in position with cotton bandages. The fingers and thumb must be left free so that the hand may be used.

flexion and extension but with slight ulnar deviation. While it is setting, the 'thenar grip' manoeuvre is repeated to mould the plaster snugly to the bones as a safeguard against redisplacement.

Immobilisation. The type of plaster depends upon individual preference. Two variations are in common use: the dorsal plaster slab (Fig. 12.19) and the complete encircling plaster (Fig. 12.20). The dorsal plaster slab covers only three-quarters of the circumference of the limb, namely the dorsum and the medial and lateral sides (Fig. 12.19): the front of the limb is left uncovered by plaster. The slab is held in position by cotton bandages. Theoretical advantages of the incomplete dorsal slab are that it may be more easily loosened if serious swelling should occur, and may thus be more safely applied immediately after reduction. In practice, the dorsal slab is often converted to a complete plaster at the first check examination 2–5 days after the injury.

In the management of a Colles's fracture it is important that the position of the fragments be checked by radiographs in two planes immediately after the reduction. These radiographs should be repeated at the time of the first check examination, because there is a risk of redisplacement as the soft-tissue swelling subsides, despite immobilisation in plaster. If the check radiographs show that redisplacement has occurred, further manipulative reduction under anaesthesia should be advised. Usually it is impossible to correct a redisplacement by manipulation if it has been allowed to persist for more than 2 weeks, so it is important to ensure that any redisplacement is detected early.

Fig. 12.20 Plaster used alternatively for a fracture of the lower end of the radius. The wrist is in a neutral position. The plaster is moulded closely to grip the lower fragment. The palm is left free beyond the proximal transverse skin crease, to allow full flexion at the metacarpophalangeal joints.

While the limb is in plaster the patient should be encouraged to use the hand freely for everyday activities, and deliberate exercises should be carried out for the fingers, elbow and shoulder.

The plaster should be retained usually for 5–6 weeks, though it may be discarded after 3 or 4 weeks in undisplaced crack fractures. Although union is far from consolidated even at 6 weeks, it is firm enough to ensure that no further displacement will occur, because the leverage acting through the short lower fragment is slight. After the plaster has been removed, a course of mobilising and muscle-strengthening exercises for the wrist and fingers should be arranged.

External fixation. Treatment by an external fixator is increasingly used as an alternative technique in younger patients with severely comminuted or displaced unstable Colles's fractures (Fig. 12.21). In these patients it is often difficult to maintain full reduction by immobilisation in plaster, but this alternative technique is only applicable when there is good bone quality to provide secure fixation for the fixator pins. A small modified external fixator is required with insertion of the distal pins either into the distal radial fragment or, alternatively, into the proximal ends of the index and middle metacarpals. This technique may also be used for maintaining the position of the fragments after corrective osteotomy for mal-union (see below).

Internal fixation. In the presence of continued instability or severe comminu-tion, particularly in the younger patient, some surgeons use limited internal

Fig. 12.21 External fixation for unstable Colles's fracture after reduction and wire fixation.

fixation of the fragments to stabilise the reduction. After closed reduction into an acceptable position, multiple percutaneous Kirschner wires or pins are inserted under radiographic control to secure the comminuted fragments. Dorsal plate fixation is less suitable for the Colles's fracture as it may interfere with extensor tendon function.

Complications

Most patients progress rapidly towards full recovery of function, and complications are infrequent considering the large number of these fractures that are treated every day. Nevertheless, the incidence of mal-union is disconcertingly high, especially in the elderly, where up to half the patients may show residual clinical deformity despite an adequate range of movement. Other complications that are seen occasionally are subluxation of the inferior radio-ulnar joint, rupture of the tendon of extensor pollicis longus, compression of the median nerve, stiffness of the fingers or shoulder from neglected use, and reflex sympathetic dystrophy (Sudeck's atrophy) of the bones of the wrist and hand.

Mal-union. It has been mentioned already that redisplacement of the fragments is liable to occur despite immobilisation in plaster, especially in the first week after reduction. If redisplacement is not detected the fragments will unite in the deformed position—that is, with backward displacement and backward tilting of the distal fragment. This is associated with a rather ugly clinical deformity, and function of the wrist is impaired.

Treatment. Each case must be considered on its merits. Often the disability is slight and can be accepted. When the deformity and impairment of function are severe enough to justify operation, correction can be achieved by an opening wedge osteotomy. The fracture site is exposed through a dorsal incision and the bone is divided at this level with an osteotome. The distal fragment is hinged downwards to restore normal alignment and the dorsal gap filled with bone graft or a bone substitute. The correction is then stabilised with percutaneous Kirschner wires or by application of an external fixator. If necessary, this operation may be combined with excision of the lower end of the ulna (see below). After internal fixation the wrist is immobilised in a plaster splint until union occurs.

Subluxation of the inferior radio-ulnar joint. This complication is caused by persistent upward displacement of the distal fragment of the radius, which is thus slightly shortened while the ulna remains of normal length. Clinically, there is pain in the region of the radio-ulnar joint, especially during active use of the wrist with a need for forearm rotation. The head of the ulna is unduly prominent at the back of the wrist, and it lies on a level with, or even below, the tip of the radial styloid process, whereas normally it lies above the level of the radial styloid (Fig. 12.22A). Wrist movements are impaired, especially adduction (ulnar deviation) and rotation.

Treatment. A minor degree of subluxation may be accepted without treatment, especially in an elderly person, but if the pain or disability is troublesome operation should be advised. A simple and reliable method is to excise the lower end of the ulna, including its head and about 3 cm of the shaft (Fig. 12.22B).

A   B

Fig. 12.22 A Subluxation of the inferior radio-ulnar joint after fracture of the lower end of the radius. There was pain over the joint, the head of the ulna was prominent, and rotation of the forearm was impaired. B After excision of the lower end of the ulna.

Rupture of extensor pollicis longus. The tendon of the extensor pollicis longus sometimes ruptures spontaneously without a preceding injury to the wrist, but the accident is much more frequent after a fracture of the lower end of the radius. The tendon is more liable to give way than its neighbours because it takes a sharp bend laterally as it leaves its groove on the back of the lower end of the radius: it therefore bears heavily against the bone as it glides to and fro with movements of the thumb, and this is the usual site of rupture. Rupture is preceded by fraying of the tendon over a length of 1–2 cm. The fracture of the lower end of the radius is not necessarily severe: indeed, the tendon seems to rupture more often after a minor crack fracture than after a major fracture with marked displacement suggesting vascular impairment as the cause.

Clinical features. The usual interval between fracture of the radius and rupture of the tendon is 4–8 weeks. Thus the symptoms may develop either while the wrist is still immobilised in plaster or soon after the plaster has been removed. In some cases the patient feels something give way at the back of the wrist, and notices immediately an inability to extend the thumb. In other cases the onset is less dramatic, the first thing to call attention to the rupture being difficulty in using the thumb. On examination there is a full range of passive movement at the thumb joints, but active extension at the interphalangeal joint is impossible and active extension at the metacarpo-phalangeal joint is greatly impaired. If the plaster has been removed there may be slight local discomfort or tenderness on palpation in the course of the tendon over the lower end of the radius.

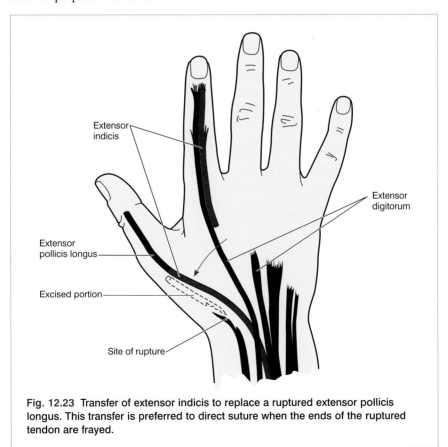

Fig. 12.23 Transfer of extensor indicis to replace a ruptured extensor pollicis longus. This transfer is preferred to direct suture when the ends of the ruptured tendon are frayed.

Treatment. Operation should be advised, but because of the extensive fraying of the tendon it is unsatisfactory to attempt end-to-end suture of the torn ends. The most reliable method is to transfer the tendon of extensor indicis to activate the distal stump of the extensor pollicis longus (Fig. 12.23). The loss of the extensor indicis does not cause significant disability, other than an impaired ability to point with the index finger.

Compression of the median nerve. Persistent backward displacement of the lower fragment of the radius leaves an anterior prominence of the lower end of the proximal fragment which may impinge against the median nerve. If there are marked symptoms of carpal tunnel compression syndrome, the nerve should be freed by open operation.

Stiffness of fingers or shoulder. If while the wrist is in plaster the patient is encouraged to use the hand and is supervised in appropriate exercises for the fingers and shoulder, stiffness from disuse will be avoided; but if the hand and shoulder are not exercised there is a serious risk of stiffness, especially in an elderly person.

Reflex sympathetic dystrophy (Sudeck's post-traumatic osteodystrophy). Reflex sympathetic dystrophy was described on page 68. It is an ill-understood condition in which the hand and fingers become markedly swollen, so that the overlying skin is stretched and glossy, and the joints become stiff. It seems to be distinct from the ordinary stiffness that may arise from disuse after a period of immobilisation in a plaster cast. A Colles's fracture is one of the most common causes of reflex sympathetic dystrophy in the upper limb, which may occur in some degree in over 30% of patients. Most patients eventually do well with conservative treatment by elevation and intensive active exercises, provided these are carried out with sufficient perseverance, though full recovery may take several months. In a few patients with refractory symptoms, more aggressive treatments may be required, including intravenous blockade with guanethidine sulphate.

FRACTURE OF THE LOWER END OF THE RADIUS WITH ANTERIOR DISPLACEMENT
(Smith's fracture, Barton's fracture)

As already mentioned (p. 178), in a small proportion of cases fracture of the lower end of the radius is associated not with the typical posterior displacement and posterior tilting of the distal fragment that characterise the Colles's fracture, but with the reverse deformity: the distal fragment is displaced forwards and tilted forwards (Fig. 12.24A). This injury is often termed Smith's[4] or Barton's[5] fracture or, loosely, reversed Colles's fracture. It is usually caused by a fall onto the back of the hand, which at the time of impact is flexed at the wrist.

---

[4]Robert W. Smith was the first Professor of Surgery in Trinity College, Dublin, and described his fracture in 1847.

[5]John Rhea Barton of Pennsylvania had described a similar injury in 1838. Since X-rays were not then available, the precise nature of these injuries is not certain, but Barton's fracture is generally regarded now as one that involves the anterior articular margin of the radius (the fracture line extending to its articular surface) whereas a Smith's fracture is entirely extra-articular.

Fig. 12.24 [A] Smith's fracture. Diagram showing typical anterior displacement and anterior tilting of the distal fragment of the radius. [B] Stabilisation of the fracture by a buttress plate screwed to the front of the proximal fragment. The flared lower half of the plate prevents the small distal fragment from slipping forward.

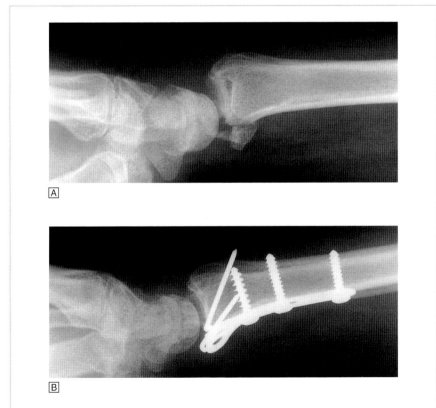

Fig. 12.25 [A] Lateral radiograph of a Barton's fracture of the distal radius with anterior displacement of the carpus and marginal fragment of the articular surface. [B] Same fracture after reduction of the articular surface and stabilisation with a buttress plate.

Treatment

For the extra-articular Smith's fracture, reduction by closed manipulation should be attempted. If this is successful, a well-moulded forearm plaster cast to include the elbow should be applied with the wrist in dorsiflexion and full supination. Weekly check radiographs are required for the first 3 weeks to ensure that redisplacement does not go undetected and the plaster retained for at least 6 weeks.

The Barton's fracture with intra-articular comminution is difficult to manage by conservative methods: reduction is often imperfect and tends to be unstable, so that redisplacement often occurs in the first 2 weeks. If an acceptable position cannot be obtained, operation is required. The lower fragment is restored to its proper position and held against redisplacement by a special buttressing plate screwed to the front of the upper fragment. The splayed lower end of the plate lies snugly against the mobile lower fragment of the radius and prevents it from slipping forward (Figs 12.24B & 12.25).

FRACTURE-SEPARATION OF THE LOWER RADIAL EPIPHYSIS

In young children fractures of the lower end of the radius are usually of the greenstick type, without much displacement. Less often an injury occurs which is the counterpart of the severely displaced Colles's fracture in adults, namely fracture-separation of the lower radial epiphysis (with or without the lower ulnar epiphysis). As the name implies, the epiphysis is separated through the epiphysial line, but a small fragment from the metaphysis is usually carried with it (Fig. 12.26). As in the typical Colles's fracture in adults, the lower fragment is usually displaced backwards. Often the displacement is severe—so much so that there may be no remaining point of contact between the separated surfaces.

Treatment

Displacement should be corrected by manipulation under anaesthesia and a plaster applied, as for fractures of the lower end of the radius in adults. Since bone healing is rapid in children, the plaster need be retained for only 3 or 4 weeks.

In some cases perfect reduction is not secured by manipulation. In that event there is no need to resort to operative reduction. Although one should always strive for accurate reduction, a somewhat imperfect position can be accepted in these young children because the deformity is rapidly effaced by the remodelling that occurs with growth.

Complications

Arrest of epiphysial growth. In crushing injuries of the epiphysial cartilage there is a risk of arrest of epiphysial growth. This is uncommon after the ordinary fracture-separation.

Elbow and forearm

Fig. 12.26 Fracture–separation of the lower radial epiphysis in a child. The distal fragment is displaced backwards and laterally Ⓐ. It has carried with it a triangular fragment of the metaphysis of the radius Ⓑ.

13 | Wrist and hand

The injuries to be described may be classified by anatomical site as follows:

Injuries of the carpus
[1] Fracture of the scaphoid bone
[2] Fractures of other carpal bones
[3] Dislocations of the lunate or other carpal bones

Injuries of the metacarpal bones and phalanges
[4] Fracture of the base of the first metacarpal
[5] Other fractures of the metacarpal bones
[6] Fractures of the phalanges
[7] Dislocations of the metacarpo-phalangeal and interphalangeal joints
Strains of the interphalangeal joints

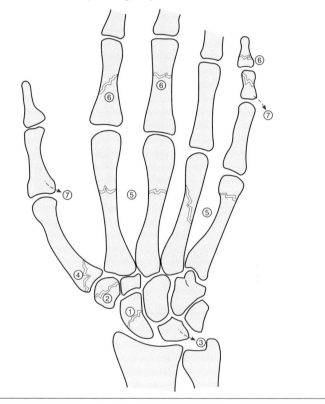

Injuries of the wrist and hand are without doubt those most commonly encountered in an accident unit. The hand in particular is so vital to the ability to earn a living that tremendous resources have been expended in studying its intricate mechanism and function—an essential background to restorative surgery. Hand surgery has now become a distinct specialty, demanding experience both of orthopaedic and of plastic surgery; skill in microsurgical techniques is also an advantage, mainly for repair of vessels and nerves, but also for replantation of severed parts. Throughout the Western world there are an increasing number of surgeons who dedicate their whole careers to the surgery of the hand.

INJURIES OF THE CARPUS

FRACTURE OF THE SCAPHOID BONE

Fracture of the scaphoid bone is common in young adults. It is not common in children or in patients of beyond middle age. The usual cause is a fall onto the outstretched hand.

The fracture nearly always occurs transversely through the middle, or waist, of the scaphoid; so the proximal and distal fragments are of about equal size (Fig. 13.1). Rarely, the fracture is through the proximal pole. Usually there is no displacement of the fragments, which lie in close apposition. If displacement does occur and is allowed to persist, it leads to a 'step' between the fragments and favours the development of degenerative arthritis.

Fractures of the distal pole through the tuberosity are rare in comparison with those of the waist of the bone, but are relatively more common in adolescent boys. They are not a clinical problem since they unite readily with minimal splintage and without long-term complications.

Fig. 13.1 A typical fracture through the waist of the scaphoid bone.

Diagnosis

Fractures of the scaphoid bone are often overlooked, either through failure to have the wrist radiographed or through failure to detect the fracture in the radiographs. In many cases the pain from the injury is slight and the patient can continue to use the hand. Thus the patient may regard the injury as a sprain and may not even consult a doctor. In other cases the doctor may be at fault because, finding little in the nature of clinical signs, the patient is not sent for radiography. In yet other instances radiographs may be obtained but the fracture is overlooked because it is not shown clearly in the initial films.

Fig. 13.2 Four different radiological views of the same scaphoid fracture (arrow).

The only safeguard against overlooking this fracture is to insist upon thorough radiographic examination in every case of wrist injury in which clinical examination shows tenderness in the scaphoid region (especially in the 'anatomical snuff-box') or impairment of wrist movements.

In radiographing a wrist for suspected fracture of the scaphoid bone the surgeon should request two oblique projections in addition to the antero-posterior and lateral projections (Fig. 13.2). Often a fracture is visible only in an oblique radiograph and gives no indication of its presence in the other films.

When the clinical features suggest fracture of the scaphoid bone but the initial radiographs give no confirmation of it, radiographic examination should be repeated after an interval of 2 weeks. A fracture may sometimes become obvious after an interval even though it was not apparent in the initial films. In the interval it is advisable to support the injured wrist in a plaster. As well as affording rest, the plaster serves the purpose of ensuring that the patient will return for re-examination.

In doubtful cases, alternative methods of diagnosis may be required when conventional radiography fails to reveal a fracture in the presence of strongly positive clinical features. The two most sensitive techniques available are magnetic resonance imaging (MRI) (Fig. 13.3), or radioisotope bone scanning, which is likely to show increased uptake of isotope at the site of any fracture.

A congenital bipartite scaphoid bone is a very rare radiological finding, but may be confused with a fracture. The bone is in two parts with a gap between them, but this is clear-cut like the other intercarpal joints, and the articulating surfaces are smooth. In cases of doubt, an MRI scan will provide a definitive diagnosis.

Treatment

The standard method of treatment in uncomplicated cases is to immobilise the wrist snugly in a plaster until the fracture is shown radiologically to be united,

Fig. 13.3 MRI scan of undisplaced scaphoid fracture (arrow).

usually in 2–3 months. Since there is usually no displacement, reduction is not required.

The plaster generally used for a scaphoid fracture is slightly more extensive than that used for a fracture of the lower end of the radius. It should extend down the thumb to the level of the interphalangeal joint, and it must be moulded firmly round the first metacarpal bone (Fig. 13.4). The palm is left free beyond the proximal skin crease to allow a full range of movement at the metacarpo-phalangeal joints of the fingers, and the thumb should be free to move at the interphalangeal joint.

In the unusual cases in which some displacement of the fragments has occurred, there is a place for operative reduction and fixation by a special compression screw (see below).

Fig. 13.4 Plaster used for fractures of the scaphoid bone. The plaster grips the first metacarpal and the proximal segment of the thumb, but the interphalangeal joint is left free. The palm is left free beyond the proximal transverse skin crease, to allow a full range of finger movements.

Complications

Fractures of the scaphoid bone, even when undisplaced, are potentially troublesome and the incidence of complications is high. The most important complications are:

- delayed union
- non-union
- avascular necrosis
- osteoarthritis.

Delayed union. In a rather high proportion of cases, fractures of the scaphoid bone unite slowly, and despite immobilisation of the wrist in plaster a fracture may be still ununited 4, 5 or even 6 months after the injury. It is uncertain whether delay in union is caused by imperfect immobilisation or by impaired blood supply to one of the fragments.

Treatment. If union has not occurred within 4 months, despite continuous rest in plaster, it is generally agreed that there is nothing to be gained by prolonging the period of immobilisation. Therefore at a point 3 or 4 weeks after the plaster has been removed and mobilising exercises commenced, a decision should be made on subsequent management. If with remobilisation the wrist causes no symptoms, there is a case for accepting the situation and deliberately ignoring the fracture. On the other hand if the wrist remains uncomfortable and much restricted in function, operation should be advised. Operation should take the form of fixation by a special compression screw, with supplementation by small sliver cancellous bone grafts if there is any gap between the fragments (Fig. 13.5).

Non-union. Although most fractures of the scaphoid bone unite readily (although sometimes slowly), there is a somewhat greater liability to non-union, with a rate of 5% in large series, compared with most other bones. In

Fig. 13.5 A case in which delayed union of a scaphoid fracture was treated by fixation by a Herbert compression screw.

Fig. 13.6 Established non-union of a fracture of the scaphoid bone. Note the well-defined fracture line and the sclerotic bone margins, suggesting a false joint between the fragments.

some cases non-union may be ascribed to imperfect immobilisation, or possibly, because the fracture is intra-articular, to the action of synovial fluid in hindering the formation of an initial fibrinous bridge between the fragments. In other cases non-union can be ascribed to impairment of the blood supply to one of the fragments. Non-union is a usual, though not inevitable, accompaniment of avascular necrosis of the proximal fragment.

When non-union has been present for a long time the fracture surfaces become rounded and sharply defined, as if a joint were forming between them (Fig. 13.6). There may also be cystic changes in one or both fragments, with some absorption of bone. Later still, the radiographs may show the beginnings of osteoarthritis with irregularity of the radio-carpal joint.

Treatment. The choice of treatment for non-union of a fracture of the scaphoid bone is influenced by the time since the original injury, the degree of functional impairment, and the presence of any secondary osteoarthritic changes.

Where symptoms are slight and disability is insignificant, the non-union may only be detected by chance on radiography of the wrist following a fresh injury to the joint. If the fracture surfaces are clean-cut and smooth, as if there were a joint between the fragments, conservative treatment in a plaster cast or orthotic brace is sometimes advocated. However, long-term radiographic studies have now shown that the development of osteoarthritic changes in the radio-carpal joint is inevitable if the non-union is allowed to persist. In these patients, as well as those with significant pain and impairment of function, the recommended treatment is internal fixation of the fracture by a compression screw. This must be supplemented by excision of any dead bone from the site of non-union and the insertion of cancellous bone graft to restore normal anatomical alignment.

In more longstanding non-union with associated partial absorption of bone or avascular changes, there is a progressive development of degenerative

Fig. 13.7 Avascular necrosis of the proximal half of a fractured scaphoid bone. The dead fragment has not shared in the disuse osteoporosis that has affected the other bones.

arthritis involving most of the carpal joints. At this stage pain, stiffness and impairment of function may become severe and require treatment for osteo-arthritis of the wrist which is described below (p. 198).

Avascular necrosis of the proximal fragment. The blood supply to the proximal fragment of the scaphoid bone is precarious after a fracture through the waist or proximal half of the bone, because the main nutrient vessels enter the distal half of the bone and must clearly be damaged by the fracture in their intraosseous course. If the remaining blood supply is inadequate the proximal fragment may die and, since it does not lie in a vascular bed, there is little chance of its becoming revascularised before irreversible changes develop which lead to crumbling of the bone. Although not common, avascular necrosis is a serious complication because it is likely to cause troublesome and permanent disability (see Fig. 13.8).

In many instances, avascular necrosis of a scaphoid fragment may be diagnosed from the radiographic appearance, because the avascular bone does not share in the general disuse osteoporosis of the carpal bones, and it therefore stands out in sharp contrast to the other bones by virtue of its relatively greater density (Fig. 13.7). This appearance is not usually manifest until about 1–3 months after the injury.

The most sensitive and specific investigation to detect early avascular changes in the bone is MRI scanning. Where available this method of imaging can also be used to monitor revascularisation of the bone following treatment.

Treatment. Avascular necrosis of the proximal fragment of the scaphoid bone commonly leads to failure of union of the fracture, but may still be amenable to treatment prior to collapse and the development of secondary degenerative arthritis. Some success has been reported using a vascularised pedicle bone graft to supplement internal fixation, though this method is only available in specialist hand surgery units. The alternative of replacing the avascular proximal fragment with a silicon rubber prosthesis gave good short-term

Fig. 13.8 Osteoarthritis of the wrist complicating the non-union of a fracture of the scaphoid bone. The marked collapse of the proximal fragment suggests that it suffered avascular necrosis.

results, but has now been abandoned because of the later development of silicone synovitis in the carpal joints. Once arthritic changes have developed no treatment can restore the wrist to normal and some permanent disability must be accepted or more radical surgical treatment undertaken.

Osteoarthritis. Osteoarthritis is a well-recognised late complication of fracture of the scaphoid bone. It tends to occur in consequence either of non-union (see p. 195) or of avascular necrosis (p. 197). It is a wear-and-tear phenomenon, initiated by damage to the articular cartilage of the scaphoid bone at the site of the fracture with consequent attrition of the cartilage on both sides of the radio-carpal joint. It may extend later to involve other carpal joints. The interval between the fracture and the development of arthritis varies from a few months to several years, according to the extent to which the scaphoid bone is disorganised, and the stresses to which the wrist is subjected.

The clinical features are pain, especially during use of the wrist, and restriction of the range of wrist movement. Radiographs show narrowing of the cartilage space and osteophytes at the joint margins, with the site of fracture still apparent (Fig. 13.8).

Treatment. Treatment is often unsatisfactory, and some permanent disability must be accepted. The choice usually lies between providing a protective wrist support (Fig. 13.9) and making the best of the situation without operation, or, in the worst examples, arthrodesis of the wrist.

Replacement arthroplasty of the wrist is not sufficiently developed at present to be recommended as an alternative to arthrodesis.

Fig. 13.9 Polythene wrist support. A splint such as this is sometimes used in the conservative treatment of osteoarthritis of the wrist.

FRACTURES OF OTHER CARPAL BONES

Apart from the scaphoid bone, the carpal bones are seldom the site of serious fractures, though isolated examples are seen from time to time. In general, the principles of treatment are like those for uncomplicated fractures of the scaphoid bone.

Flake fracture of the triquetral bone

This is a minor chip fracture often caused by a fall on the hand in hyperflexion or hyperextension. There is pain at the back of the wrist, and the lateral radiograph shows a small flake of bone detached from the dorsal surface of the triquetrum (Fig. 13.10). Only symptomatic treatment is required, usually with 3 weeks of plaster immobilisation to relieve pain, and thereafter full function is quickly restored.

Kienböck's disease of the lunate bone

This uncommon condition may be confused with a fracture of the lunate when radiographs are taken of a painful swollen wrist. These show a squashed or flattened bone in which the substance has become soft, granular and fragmented. The aetiology of the condition is unknown, but may result from repeated microtrauma causing interference with the blood supply of the bone. Though this form of avascular necrosis occurs in adults, it resembles the osteochondritis of childhood and is described more fully in orthopaedic textbooks. In the absence of treatment the deformity and irregularity of the articular surface of the bone quickly lead to severe osteoarthritis.

Dislocation of the carpal bones

Complete dislocation of the wrist—that is, dislocation of the carpus as a whole from the radius—is very uncommon and need not be described here. Various types of incomplete carpal dislocation are recognised, in which one or more of the carpal bones are displaced, and the dislocation may be associated with a fracture. The injuries seen most frequently are (1) dislocation of the lunate bone and (2) perilunar dislocation of the carpus.

Fig. 13.10 Flake fracture (arrow) on dorsum of triquetrum.

Dislocation of the lunate bone

It is surprising that a bone that nestles so snugly between its neighbours, and which has strong ligamentous attachments, should be liable to dislocation through a fall onto the hand. However, the lunate bone is somewhat wedge-shaped with its base anteriorly, and with the hand extended in a fall the bone may be squeezed out from between the capitate bone and the radius. The displacement in a lateral radiograph is characteristic: the lunate bone lies at the front of the wrist and it is rotated through 90° or more on a horizontal axis so that its concave lower articular surface faces forwards (Figs 13.11A & C). For the lunate bone to reach this position it is clear that its posterior ligamentous attachments must be torn, so that it hinges on the anterior ligaments.

Treatment

Closed reduction by manipulation should be attempted under anaesthesia. Strong traction is first applied to the hand to open up the space for the lunate bone. Direct pressure is then applied over the displaced bone and it may pop back into position. If so, the position should be stabilised with percutaneous Kirschner wires before a plaster is applied to avoid redisplacement. The plaster and wires are retained for 4 weeks before active mobilising exercises are begun.

In many cases where there has been delay in diagnosis manipulation may be unsuccessful. In that event the bone should be replaced by operation, with supplementary stabilisation of the carpus with Kirschner wires. In old neglected cases in which the dislocation has been present for a long time it may be necessary to excise the bone rather than attempt to replace it. In such a case, permanent impairment of wrist function is inevitable.

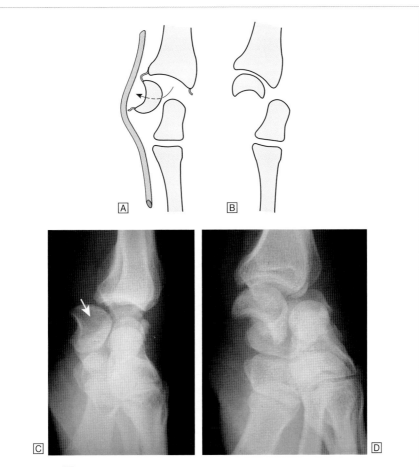

Fig. 13.11 [A] Dislocation of the lunate bone. Note the position of the median nerve, which may suffer injury. [B] Perilunar dislocation of the carpus. This is basically the same injury as dislocation of the lunate bone, in that the remainder of the carpus is separated from the lunate bone. The two may thus be regarded as variations of the same injury. [C] Radiograph of typical lunate dislocation. [D] Radiograph of perilunar dislocation of carpus.

Complications

The blood supply of the displaced lunate bone is precarious because many of its soft-tissue attachments are torn; so there is a risk of avascular necrosis and later of osteoarthritis. There is also a risk of injury to the median nerve from direct pressure of the displaced bone (Fig 13.11A).

Avascular necrosis. After a dislocated lunate bone has been replaced—whether by manipulation or operation—its condition should be observed by radiography or MRI scanning at 2-monthly intervals. If its blood supply is inadequate, signs of avascular necrosis may appear within 1–4 months, though this is surprisingly uncommon.

Osteoarthritis. Osteoarthritis will occur inevitably if the lunate bone is avascular and if it is not excised. When osteoarthritis is already established it is too late to hope for improvement from excision of the bone. Treatment should be conservative at first—for instance, by a leather or plastic wrist support (Fig. 13.9)—but if the disability becomes severe the only satisfactory treatment is by arthrodesis of the wrist.

Injury to median nerve. The median nerve is liable to be trapped between the displaced lunate bone and the flexor retinaculum. If the nerve is injured there will be signs of sensory and motor impairment in the median distribution in the hand. If these are present, the nerve must be decompressed as soon as possible by reduction of the lunate dislocation or, in long-standing cases, by excision of the lunate bone. At the same time the flexor retinaculum should be divided to decompress the carpal tunnel.

Dislocation of the lunate and half scaphoid

This is exactly the same injury as that just described except that the displaced lunate bone carries with it the adjacent (proximal) half of the scaphoid bone, which is fractured into two roughly equal halves through its waist. The principles of treatment are the same. The scaphoid fracture will require fixation with a screw or Kirschner wire if the fragments are not in exact apposition after reduction of the dislocation (see p. 195).

Perilunar dislocation of the carpus

In this injury the whole carpus is dislocated backwards except for the lunate bone, which remains in normal relationship with the radius (Fig. 13.11B&D).

So far as the relationship between the lunate bone and the rest of the carpus is concerned, there is no difference between this injury and a dislocation of the lunate bone (Figs 13.11A & C). Indeed, a perilunar dislocation of the carpus is sometimes converted into a dislocation of the lunate bone during attempted reduction. The treatment by closed or open reduction with Kirschner wire fixation is the same as for isolated dislocation of the lunate.

Trans-scapho-perilunar dislocation of the carpus

This is exactly the same injury as perilunar dislocation of the carpus except that the scaphoid bone is fractured and its proximal half remains attached to the lunate bone, in normal relationship with the radius.

INJURIES OF THE METACARPAL BONES AND PHALANGES

A preliminary note is in order here on the matter of immobilisation of the fingers after fracture. It has been found that the metacarpo-phalangeal joints tend to stiffen if they are held extended, whereas the reverse is the case with the interphalangeal joints: they tend to stiffen most if held flexed. In general, therefore, if immobilisation is required the aim should be to splint the metacarpo-phalangeal joints in about 70° of flexion, and the interphalangeal joints in a position close to full extension (Fig. 13.12). There are few exceptions to this rule, but of course each case must be considered on its merits.

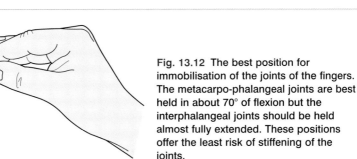

Fig. 13.12 The best position for immobilisation of the joints of the fingers. The metacarpo-phalangeal joints are best held in about 70° of flexion but the interphalangeal joints should be held almost fully extended. These positions offer the least risk of stiffening of the joints.

It should also be borne in mind that fingers tolerate immobilisation badly, even when the above rule is observed. To immobilise an injured finger for a long time is to court disaster in the form of prolonged or even permanent stiffness. It should be regarded as a sound working rule that a fractured finger should never be immobilised for more than 3 weeks. After that time, active exercises must be begun, irrespective of the condition of the fracture.

FRACTURE OF THE BASE OF THE FIRST METACARPAL BONE

A fracture of the base of the first metacarpal bone is usually sustained from forced abduction of the thumb, or longitudinal violence applied by a blow, as in boxing. Clinically there is local tenderness distal to the anatomical snuff box, unlike a scaphoid fracture, and this may be accompanied by deformity.

Pathology

There are two distinct types of this injury (Fig. 13.13): (1) a transverse or short oblique fracture across the base of the metacarpal, but not entering the joint and (2) an oblique fracture entering the carpo-metacarpal joint at about the middle

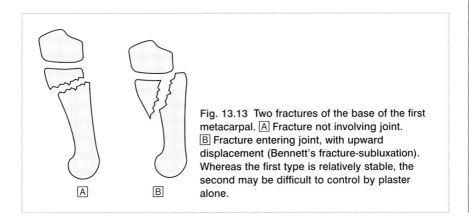

Fig. 13.13 Two fractures of the base of the first metacarpal. A Fracture not involving joint. B Fracture entering joint, with upward displacement (Bennett's fracture-subluxation). Whereas the first type is relatively stable, the second may be difficult to control by plaster alone.

Fig. 13.14 A Intra-articular Bennett's fracture-subluxation. Note the proximal and lateral displacement of the distal or main fragment. B Extra-articular fracture at base of thumb metacarpal.

of the articular surface (Bennett's fracture-subluxation[1]). The second type is the more serious, because unless a smooth joint surface can be restored there is a risk of the later development of osteoarthritis. When the fracture is oblique there is a strong tendency for the large distal fragment to be displaced backwards and upwards upon the small proximal fragment which remains in articulation with the trapezium (Figs 13.13B & 13.14A). This displacement results from the pull of the abductor pollicis longus tendon.

Treatment

Displacement can nearly always be reduced by manipulation under anaesthesia, but it is often difficult, in the oblique Bennett fracture, to maintain the reduction. An attempt should be made to do this by applying a well-moulded plaster, which should include the forearm and wrist and should hold the thumb metacarpal well extended at the carpo-metacarpal joint. Check radiographs should be taken twice during the first week to determine whether a good position has been maintained.

Slight loss of position matters little in the case of a fracture that does not involve the joint, but full reduction should be the aim if the joint surface is involved. In the majority of intra-articular fractures, therefore, operation should be advised. At operation it may be feasible to fix the fragments together with a small screw (Fig. 13.15A). If not, an alternative method is by the use of a percutaneous Kirschner wire after the fracture is first reduced by traction combined with thumb pressure against the displaced base of the metacarpal. The Kirschner wire is driven obliquely through the base of the metacarpal into the trapezium (Fig. 13.15B). After fixation by either method a well-fitting plaster should be retained for 4–6 weeks.

---

[1] Edward Hallaran Bennett was Professor of Surgery at Trinity College, Dublin, and described this injury in 1882. His report pre-dated radiology and was based on bone pathology specimens and clinical examination.

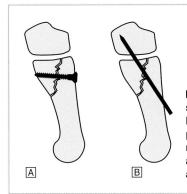

Fig. 13.15 Two methods of stabilising a fracture-subluxation of the base of the first metacarpal bone. A Fixation by a screw. B Stabilisation by percutaneous pin driven through the base of the metacarpal into the trapezium. Operation is advised only when reduction cannot be held by a plaster.

Complications

Osteoarthritis. The risk of osteoarthritis has been mentioned already. It will occur only after a fracture that has damaged the joint surface and left it irregular. It may occasionally be a cause of troublesome disability if the hand is used for heavy work. Exceptionally it may demand operation, either arthrodesis of the trapezio-metacarpal joint or, more often, excision of the trapezium.

OTHER FRACTURES OF THE METACARPAL BONES

- Fractures of the metacarpal bones are fairly common at all ages. The most common causes are a fall onto the hand or a blow on the knuckles as in boxing. These fractures may be classified according to site, as follows:
- Fracture through the base of the metacarpal (Fig. 13.16A). This is usually transverse and undisplaced.

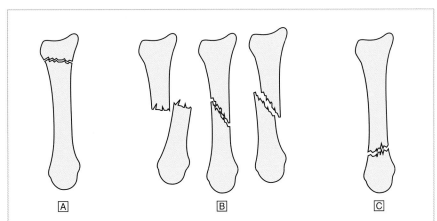

Fig. 13.16 Fractures of metacarpal bones. The diagrams show the three sites of fracture—A base, B shaft, and C neck. In the absence of displacement treatment is hardly necessary. Severe displacement, shortening or angulation demands correction, if necessary by operation.

Fig. 13.17 A common metacarpal fracture that may be difficult to treat. The fracture is through the neck of the fifth metacarpal and the head of the bone is tilted forwards into flexion.

- Fracture through the shaft. This may be transverse or oblique. A transverse fracture may be undisplaced, or there may be wide separation with overlap of the fragments (Fig. 13.16B). An oblique fracture tends to allow telescoping with consequent shortening and recession of the knuckle (Fig. 13.16B).
- Fracture through the neck of the metacarpal. This may be undisplaced (Fig. 13.16C), but, particularly in the fifth metacarpal, there may be marked forward tilting of the distal fragment (Fig. 13.17).

Treatment

The treatment depends upon the degree of displacement. There are thus two groups to be considered: those in which the existing position is acceptable, and those in which the position cannot be accepted.

Undisplaced fractures (including those with acceptable displacement). These comprise a large proportion of the total. The position is stable, and treatment is simple—indeed sound union and perfect recovery of function may be expected without treatment of any kind, but simply with active use of the hand. Over-treatment should therefore be avoided. It is nevertheless wise in some cases to provide temporary support for relief of pain and apprehension. A common method is to apply a light dorsal plaster slab for 3 weeks. Finger movements and active use of the hand must be encouraged from the beginning.

Displaced fractures. In the less common case with unacceptable displacement or angulation, reduction of displacement and maintenance of the correction are required. Whether this can be achieved by manual reduction and external splintage, or whether operation will be required, depends on the nature of the individual fracture.

In transverse fractures displacement with loss of end-to-end apposition may result in overlap and necessitate open reduction with intramedullary wire or miniature plate fixation.

In the long oblique fracture telescoping with rotational malalignment is more likely to produce shortening with an unsightly recession of the knuckle. Manual traction will reduce the displacement but recurrence is common unless fixation is secured with a transfixion wire or small fragment screws. When multiple metacarpal fractures occur as a result of more severe crush injuries of the hand, open reduction and more stable internal fixation is required with small fragment plates.

An isolated displaced fracture of the neck of the fifth metacarpal (Fig. 13.17) occurs fairly commonly as the `boxer's fracture'. Reduction by dorsal displacement of the distal fragment is relatively easy to achieve, but difficult to maintain. The fracture will still heal quickly in 3–4 weeks without loss of function, but may leave an unsightly cosmetic deformity. However, surgical fixation with a Kirschner wire is only required when the angulation is greater than 40°.

FRACTURES OF THE PHALANGES

The various patterns of fracture that are met with in the phalanges of the fingers are shown in Figure 13.18A.

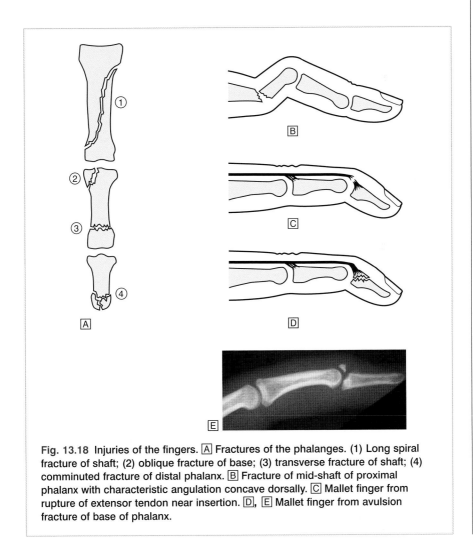

Fig. 13.18 Injuries of the fingers. Ⓐ Fractures of the phalanges. (1) Long spiral fracture of shaft; (2) oblique fracture of base; (3) transverse fracture of shaft; (4) comminuted fracture of distal phalanx. Ⓑ Fracture of mid-shaft of proximal phalanx with characteristic angulation concave dorsally. Ⓒ Mallet finger from rupture of extensor tendon near insertion. Ⓓ, Ⓔ Mallet finger from avulsion fracture of base of phalanx.

Treatment

The advice relating to immobilisation of the finger joints set out on p. 203 should be noted at this point also. Immobilisation should be kept to a minimum. Nearly all phalangeal fractures will proceed to bony union whether they are splinted or not; so the main purposes of splintage are to prevent redisplacement of fractures that have required reduction, and to relieve pain. Both these purposes will often have been achieved within 2 or 3 weeks, and therefore with few exceptions there is no further need for splintage after that time.

Undisplaced fractures of the shaft. The fragments are held together by the periosteal sheath. There is no fear of displacement. Treatment is unnecessary except to relieve pain. A simple method of affording support without immobilisation is to bind the phalanges of the injured finger lightly to the corresponding segments of an adjacent normal finger with adhesive strapping. The sound finger thus acts to support the injured one, the so-called 'buddy splintage'.

Displaced fractures and fractures involving joint surfaces. An attempt should be made to reduce the displacement by manipulation and, if this is successful, to hold the position by a simple malleable splint. Immobilisation should be discontinued in favour of active exercises after not more than 3 weeks. Figure 13.18B shows an example.

If displacement cannot be controlled in this way, operation may be required. The fragments may be held in position by transfixion with two Kirschner wires inserted percutaneously after manipulation, or after open reduction. Small fragments may often be repositioned and held by a wire stitch anchored through fine drill holes.

Comminuted fractures of distal phalanx. The pulp or the nail bed may be torn, and the nail may often separate. The fracture should be ignored and attention directed solely to the soft-tissue injury, for which dry dressings covered by protective soft wool and a cotton bandage will usually be required.

Mallet finger
(Baseball finger)

Sudden passive flexion of the distal interphalangeal joint (as by a ball striking the tip of the finger) may rupture the extensor tendon at the point of its insertion into the base of the distal phalanx (Fig. 13.18C). Sometimes a fragment of bone is avulsed from the phalanx (Figs 13.18D & E). Clinically, the distal interphalangeal joint rests in moderate flexion and cannot be actively extended. In the early stages there is tenderness over the site of avulsion.

Treatment

Tendon avulsion, with or without a small bone fragment, is treated by uninterrupted splintage in the fully straight position for 6 weeks. Immobilisation is confined to the distal interphalangeal joints, the proximal joint being left free. Healing may occur with a small residual extensor lag, but this is functionally acceptable.

If a larger fragment of bone has been avulsed the displacement may be reduced at operation and the fragment held in position by a Kirschner wire passed through the distal phalanx and the reduced fragment, and across the joint to hold it fully extended; or alternatively the fragment may be stabilised by a fine wire stitch passed through the tendon close to the bone fragment and anchored to the base of the phalanx through fine drill holes.

DISLOCATIONS OF THE METACARPO-PHALANGEAL AND INTERPHALANGEAL JOINTS

Most dislocations of the finger and thumb joints are caused by forced hyperextension. The distal segment is usually displaced backwards from the proximal (Fig. 13.19).

Treatment

The dislocation should be reduced with the least possible delay. Reduction is usually effected easily by pulling upon the digit and applying direct pressure over the base of the displaced phalanx. This can often be done without anaesthesia. Radiographs should be taken to check the reduction. Immobilisation is not required, and active movements of the joint should be encouraged from an early stage.

'Button-hole' injuries. Sometimes in metacarpo-phalangeal dislocations the head of the metacarpal bone is driven forwards through a rent in the front of the capsule at the same time as the phalanx is dislocated backwards. In this event manipulative reduction may be impossible and operation is required. The capsular slit is enlarged sufficiently to allow it to be hooked back over the metacarpal head.

STRAINS OF THE INTERPHALANGEAL JOINTS

Strains of the interphalangeal joints are notorious for their chronicity. The joint may remain swollen and painful for as long as 6 or 9 months after a relatively minor injury. Yet there is little or no restriction of movement and full recovery occurs eventually.

The causative injury is usually an angulation force with incomplete disruption of the medial or lateral ligament and of the joint capsule. The consequent periarticular thickening causes a characteristic fusiform swelling about the

Fig. 13.19 A typical dislocation of a finger. The middle phalanx is displaced backwards upon the proximal.

joint. Radiographs may show no bone injury, but sometimes a tiny flake of bone is avulsed at the point of attachment of the capsule.

Treatment

In mild cases treatment is unnecessary. If pain is severe the finger may be supported by a light bandage or strapping to the adjacent digit for a week before active movements are begun. The tendency to slow rather than rapid recovery should be explained to the patient.

CLASSIFICATION

FRACTURES OF THE PELVIS

A. Isolated fractures—stable with no disruption of the pelvic ring
   [1] Fracture of superior ischio-pubic ramus
   [2] Fracture of inferior ischio-pubic ramus
   [3] Fracture entering wall of acetabulum
   [4] Fracture of wing of ilium
   [5] Avulsion fractures of anterior inferior iliac spine, anterior superior iliac spine, or ischial tuberosity.

B. Fractures with disruption of the pelvic ring—unstable
   [1] Combination of anterior and posterior fractures of the pelvic ring
   [2] Disruption of pubic symphysis and posterior sacro-iliac joint

Fractures of the pelvis are relatively uncommon and present problems of management only if they cause instability of the bony ring of the pelvis, or complications from damage to the pelvic contents.

Injuries of the hip joint itself are much less common than fractures of the upper end of the femur and femoral neck, which are also included in this chapter for anatomical convenience.

ISOLATED FRACTURES

Any part of the pelvis may be affected. The most common fractures occur through the superior or inferior ischio-pubic ramus, or through both rami: these may be combined with a fracture through the acetabulum, but in the absence of displacement they may be included in this group of relatively benign fractures. Fractures of the pubic rami often occur in elderly patients as a result of minor falls on the side. The patient may be unable to stand because of pain in the hip area and a fracture of the proximal femur may be suspected. An X-ray of the pelvis will identify the fracture of the ischio-pubic ramus (Fig. 14.1) as the true source of the pain. This injury should be regarded as a fragility fracture and the patient investigated and treated for any underlying osteoporosis.

Avulsion fractures are increasingly common in adolescents and professional athletes as a result of sudden violent contraction of a muscle with partial or complete separation of its bony insertion. The commoner sites are the rectus femoris insertion at the anterior inferior spine, the hamstrings at the ischial ramus, and the sartorious at the anterior superior spine.

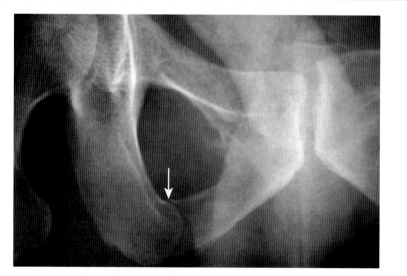

Fig. 14.1 Fracture of the ischio-pubic ramus (arrow).

Treatment

For many of these injuries no special treatment is needed, except to relieve pain. A short period of bed rest followed by protected weight-bearing with a walking aid is usually sufficient. Exercises for the lower limb should be encouraged from the beginning.

In the occasional case of complete avulsion fracture, an operation may be required to fix back the bone fragment to allow the patient to return to full sporting activity.

Complications

Complications are uncommon in these relatively minor fractures of the pelvis. Occasionally the bladder or urethra may be damaged by a sharp fragment of bone, displaced from the ischio-pubic ramus in more violent direct injuries.

FRACTURES WITH DISRUPTION OF THE PELVIC RING

The pelvic ring is composed of the sacrum and the two innominate bones. Disruption of the ring can occur only if there are fractures or dislocations at two points approximately opposite one another. Thus a fracture in the anterior half of the ring with separation of the fragments must be associated with an injury in the posterior half of the ring. In most cases of this type the anterior injury takes the form of a fracture through both ischio-pubic rami with separation, or of disruption of the symphysis pubis (Fig. 14.2). The posterior injury is usually a dislocation or subluxation of the sacro-iliac joint, or a fracture through the ilium or the lateral mass (ala) of the sacrum near the sacro-iliac joint. Displacement between the two halves of the pelvis is usually slight, but it may be

Fig. 14.2 Disruption of the symphysis pubis. In this case the posterior injury was a subluxation of the left sacro-iliac joint.

severe, with the innominate bone displaced markedly upwards in relation to the sacrum.

These severe pelvic fractures are usually caused by direct injury, or by violence transmitted longitudinally through the femur. The mechanism of the injury may be (1) antero-posterior crushing; (2) compression from side to side or (3) a vertical shearing force, which may cause marked displacement of one half of the pelvis.

Treatment

Major fractures of the pelvis present difficult problems of management, especially when the acetabulum is involved or when there is disruption of a sacro-iliac joint. In patients who are otherwise fit, every effort should be made to restore the normal anatomy, if necessary by operation. Severe shock is often a feature of major fractures of the pelvis, and it may demand strenuous resuscitative measures. The surgeon should be alert to the possibility of massive internal haemorrhage from rupture of a major vessel. Persistent retroperitoneal bleeding may demand operation for ligature of the internal iliac artery. Where sophisticated radiological services are available, it may be possible to identify the site of haemorrhage by arteriography and to secure local haemostasis by injecting a fibrin clot after selective catheterisation.

If displacement is slight, all that is required is rest in bed until the two halves of the pelvis become united reasonably firmly, usually a matter of 4–6 weeks. During the period of rest, exercises for the lower limbs should be carried out daily to keep the joints mobile and the muscles active.

Disruption of the symphysis pubis. It is important that the displacement be fully reduced and the position stabilised without delay, because the urethra, if not already ruptured, is in jeopardy. It is sometimes possible to reduce the displacement by manual pressure on both iliac crests with the patient in the recumbent position and to provide temporary stabilisation with crossed pelvic slings. A more reliable method is by the application of an external fixation frame on the anterior aspect of the pelvis. Multiple threaded pins are inserted at two sites in the anterior part of the wing of the ilium on each side, and attached by clamps to adjustable transverse metal bars to form a rectangular frame (Fig. 14.3). This has the additional advantages of controlling bleeding and pain, easing nursing care, and allowing access to the abdomen for laparotomy if required.

An alternative method is to use internal fixation of the pubic rami with contoured plates and screws. This should only be considered when laparotomy is required for visceral injury, or following transfer to a specialist trauma centre.

Upward displacement of the half pelvis. In disruption injuries from a severe shearing force one innominate bone may be displaced markedly upwards. In that event an attempt should be made to reduce the displacement by heavy weight traction applied through a femoral or a tibial pin (see Fig. 15.3, p. 241). When reduction has been achieved, the position may be held by screws driven across the sacro-iliac joint.

Complications

Rupture of the bladder. The bladder may be torn open in disruptions of the symphysis pubis or it may be penetrated by a spike of bone. The rupture is

Fig. 14.3 External pelvic fixation. A method of holding a disrupted pubic symphysis reduced by pins driven into the iliac bone on each side and joined by articulated transverse bars (diagrammatic).

usually extraperitoneal, and urine is extravasated into the perivesical space. The patient is shocked: he or she has a desire to pass urine but is unable to do so. A catheter passes easily into the bladder but only a few drops of blood-stained fluid escape. Emergency urethrography will distinguish this injury from rupture of the urethra.

Treatment. Urgent operation is required, and whenever possible it should be undertaken by a urological surgeon. The principles of treatment are: (1) to suture the rent, (2) to drain the bladder and (3) to drain the perivesical space.

Rupture of the urethra. This also is most common in cases of wide disruption of the symphysis pubis. The rupture is usually in the membranous part. Extravasation will occur into the perineum if the patient attempts to pass urine. If a ruptured urethra is suspected, the patient should be warned not to attempt to pass urine. It will be impossible to pass a catheter into the bladder, and there may be a little blood at the meatus.

Treatment. Urgent operation is required, and the cooperation of a urological surgeon should be sought. The principles of treatment are to: (1) to identify the torn ends of the urethra through incisions in the perineum and, if necessary, in the bladder; (2) to suture the ends, if necessary over a catheter passed into the bladder; (3) to drain the bladder suprapubically and (4) to close the perineal wound with drainage.

Injury to the rectum or vagina. There may be disruption of the perineum, with damage to the rectum or vagina. These injuries are uncommon, and need not be considered fully here.

Injury to a major blood vessel. Rarely the common iliac artery or one of its branches may be ruptured or damaged by a spike of bone. In the case of a main vessel, with threat to the viability of the limb, the torn ends of the vessel should be sutured or, if direct suture is impracticable, continuity may be restored by a vein graft. Severance of a smaller artery with formation of a massive haematoma may necessitate arteriography to embolise the vessel itself or, occasionally, it may be expedient to ligate the internal iliac artery proximal to the site of bleeding.

Injury to nerves. In a case of major disruption of the pelvic ring with marked upward displacement of the half pelvis, it is common for nerves of the lumbo-sacral plexus to be injured. In some of these cases there is a vertical fracture of the sacrum with wide displacement, and individual nerves may be damaged as they lie within the sacral foramina. In other cases the disruption occurs through the sacro-iliac joint, and then presumably the nerve trunks may be damaged by stretching. Although these nerve injuries may sometimes fall within the groups of neurapraxia or axonotmesis and show full or partial recovery, in most cases the injury is irrecoverable and the consequent weakness or paralysis—which may be of patchy distribution—is permanent. There may also be disturbance of sexual function.

Involvement of the acetabulum with subsequent osteoarthritis. A fracture extending into the acetabulum may leave the articular surface roughened. The increased wear-and-tear may then lead gradually to the development of osteoarthritis of the hip. Fractures involving the acetabulum are considered further in the following section.

DISLOCATIONS AND FRACTURE–DISLOCATIONS OF THE HIP

Only three types of dislocation and fracture–dislocation of the hip need be considered:

1. posterior dislocation or fracture–dislocation
2. anterior dislocation
3. central fracture–dislocation.

All these injuries are uncommon when compared, for example, with dislocation of the shoulder. Of the three types, the posterior dislocation is the most common.

Diagnosis

It is surprising, but nevertheless true, that a dislocation or fracture–dislocation of the hip has often been overlooked even by experienced surgeons. This grave mistake is liable to be made when there are other serious injuries in the same limb, particularly a fracture of the shaft of the femur. In such a case the symptoms and signs of the shaft fracture may so overshadow those of the hip injury that neither the patient's nor the surgeon's attention is drawn to the hip. The essential safeguards against this error are, firstly, to insist always on a full clinical survey of the whole body in cases of major injury; and, secondly, to make sure that the radiographs in every case of fractured femoral shaft take in the whole length of the bone and include the hip joint.

POSTERIOR DISLOCATION AND FRACTURE–DISLOCATION

The femoral head is forced out of the back of the acetabulum by violence applied along the shaft of the femur while the hip is flexed or semiflexed (Fig. 14.4A). The injury often occurs as a result of a motor accident in which the

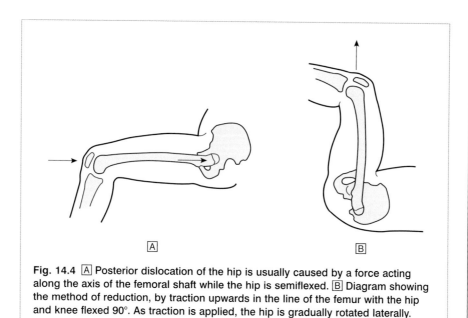

Fig. 14.4 [A] Posterior dislocation of the hip is usually caused by a force acting along the axis of the femoral shaft while the hip is semiflexed. [B] Diagram showing the method of reduction, by traction upwards in the line of the femur with the hip and knee flexed 90°. As traction is applied, the hip is gradually rotated laterally.

occupant of a car involved in a collision is thrown forwards and strikes the front of the flexed knee against a part of the bodywork. Another common cause is a motor-cycle crash.

In about half the cases of posterior dislocation of the hip, the head of the femur carries with it a small or large fragment of bone from the rim of the acetabulum (fracture–dislocation; see Fig. 14.6). It should be noted that the sciatic nerve is almost directly in the path of displacement and may easily be damaged.

Clinical features

To remember the clinical deformity it is easiest to think of the greater trochanter as being held more or less in its normal position by the attached muscles—as if by guy ropes—and forming the centre of a new vertical axis about which the femoral head may swing forwards or backwards (Fig. 14.5). Thus in a posterior dislocation the femur—and with it the whole lower limb—is rotated medially as well as being displaced upwards (Fig. 14.5). There will be true shortening of the limb, perhaps by 2 or 3 cm. Radiographs will confirm the dislocation (Fig. 14.6) and show whether or not there is an associated fracture. Careful examination should always be made for signs of injury to the sciatic nerve.

Treatment

The dislocation should be reduced under general anaesthesia as soon as possible. Reduction is usually effected without difficulty by pulling longitudinally upon the femur while the hip is flexed to a right angle and rotated laterally.

Technique. The patient is placed supine, preferably on the floor or on a low table, and an assistant grasps the pelvis firmly through the iliac crests. The surgeon flexes the hip and knee to a right angle so that the line of the femur

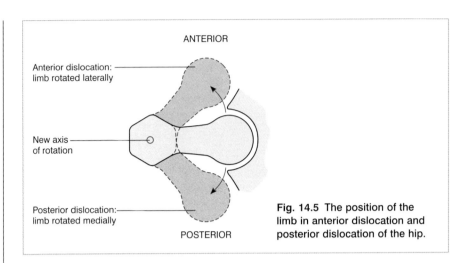

ANTERIOR

Anterior dislocation:
limb rotated laterally

New axis
of rotation

Posterior dislocation:
limb rotated medially

POSTERIOR

Fig. 14.5 The position of the limb in anterior dislocation and posterior dislocation of the hip.

Fig. 14.6 Posterior dislocation of the left hip sustained in a motor-cycle crash with marginal acetabular fracture (arrow).

points vertically upwards, and then pulls the thigh steadily upwards, at the same time gradually rotating the femur laterally (Fig. 14.4B).

After the dislocation has been reduced the limb is supported from a beam, with light traction, for 3–6 weeks. Meanwhile mobilising exercises for the hip and knee are begun after a few days and are gradually intensified.

Persistent displacement of an acetabular fragment. A small marginal fragment from the acetabulum will usually fall back into place when the dislocation is reduced. If a large acetabular fragment remains unreduced, operation is required. The fragment is exposed through a posterior incision, reduced under direct vision, and fixed in place by a screw or small plate. It is essential that full anatomical reduction of the displaced fragment be achieved. Any remaining 'step' or irregularity of the acetabular surface will predispose to later osteoarthritis.

Complications
These are: (1) injury to the sciatic nerve, (2) damage to the femoral head, (3) avascular necrosis of the femoral head, (4) post-traumatic ossification and (5) osteoarthritis.

Injury to the sciatic nerve. The nerve is vulnerable to injury where it lies behind the posterior wall of the acetabulum. It may be damaged in a dislocation without fracture of the acetabulum, but it is particularly liable to severe injury when a large fragment of the acetabular wall is driven backwards with the head of the femur. The nerve lesion is usually a neurapraxia or an axonotmesis (p. 63), but it may be virtually a complete division (neurotmesis).

Treatment. Pressure upon the nerve must be relieved at the earliest moment by reduction of the dislocation and replacement of displaced bone fragments, if necessary by operation. Thereafter treatment is usually expectant at first, as for other closed nerve injuries (p. 64), but if operation has to be undertaken to replace a large acetabular fragment the opportunity should be taken to examine the nerve at the same time.

Prognosis. The outlook for recovery is good after a minor nerve lesion of the type classed as neurapraxia. But after severe injuries of the sciatic nerve at this high level the prognosis for recovery of good muscle power is poor because of the length to be regenerated and the likelihood that the distal muscles will have suffered irreversible changes before they are reinnervated. The prognosis for sensory recovery is also doubtful.

Damage to the femoral head. Rarely, the femoral head may be split by forcible impact against the acetabular margin. More often the damage is not obvious radiologically and may consist in severe bruising of the articular cartilage or subclinical fracture of the subchondral bone or of trabeculae of the femoral head. Such injury may lead to degenerative arthritis in later life.

Avascular necrosis of the femoral head. The general subject of avascular necrosis was discussed on page 57. There is a rather high incidence of avascular necrosis of the femoral head after posterior dislocation of the hip: the incidence may be higher when there has been delay in reduction, probably in the order of 15–20%. The complication is presumably caused by damage to blood vessels in the ligament of the femoral head (ligamentum teres) and in the capsule, which may be extensively torn. In the course of several months the avascular head gradually collapses, wholly or in part, and osteoarthritis of the hip is the inevitable sequel (Fig. 14.7).

Post-traumatic ossification. Occasionally a mass of new bone forms about the hip, from ossification in the haematoma that collects beneath the stripped-up periosteum and capsule (so-called myositis ossificans, see p. 67).

Osteoarthritis. After a dislocation of the hip, osteoarthritis may arise from three distinct causes: avascular necrosis of the femoral head (see above), roughening of the acetabulum from a fracture involving its articular surface, and damage to the femoral head or its articular cartilage.

When avascular necrosis is responsible, the features of osteoarthritis usually begin to be evident within a few months of the dislocation, though often there is a latent period of up to a year or more before arthritis becomes incapacitating.

When osteoarthritis follows roughening of the acetabulum consequent upon a fracture, or when it follows damage to the femoral head, it tends to develop more slowly; indeed, if the damage has been slight, many years may elapse before the arthritis becomes troublesome.

Fig. 14.7 Marked irregularity and partial collapse of the femoral head (arrow) a year and a half after posterior dislocation of the hip. The changes suggest that part of the femoral head suffered avascular necrosis from damage to its blood supply at the time of the injury.

ANTERIOR DISLOCATION

Anterior dislocation of the hip is much less common than posterior dislocation. Indeed, it is a very uncommon injury. It is caused by forced abduction and lateral rotation of the limb, usually in a violent injury such as a motor accident or aircraft crash. There is not usually an associated fracture of the acetabular margin. **Clinically**, the limb rests in marked lateral rotation (Fig. 14.5).

Treatment
Reduction under anaesthesia is effected by strong traction upon the limb combined with medial rotation. Thereafter, treatment is the same as for posterior dislocation.

Complications
There is not the same risk of damage to the sciatic nerve as there is in posterior dislocations, but the femoral nerve and artery may be compressed, and the risk of osteoarthritis from avascular necrosis is the same.

CENTRAL FRACTURE–DISLOCATION

In central fracture–dislocation of the hip the femoral head is driven through the medial wall, or 'floor', of the acetabulum towards the pelvic cavity. It differs from anterior and posterior dislocations in that the capsule remains intact, but there is inevitably a fracture of the acetabulum, usually with much comminution.

Central fracture–dislocation is caused by a heavy lateral blow upon the femur, as in a fall from a height onto the side or a crushing injury, or it may be caused by a longitudinal force acting upon the femur (as from a blow upon the flexed knee) while the hip is abducted. The degree of displacement varies with

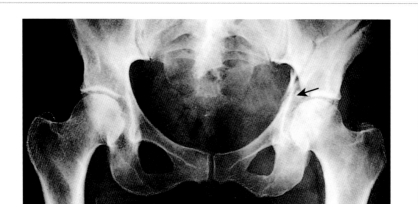

Fig. 14.8 Fracture of the acetabulum with slight medial displacement of the femoral head and acetabular floor. The main part of the weight-bearing surface of the acetabulum is intact. With traction, or failing that by operation, a reasonably smooth acetabular surface may be restored, but there is nevertheless a serious risk that osteoarthritis will develop later.

the severity of the violence. Thus in the minor varieties of the injury the femoral head and the medial wall of the acetabulum may be displaced inwards by only a few millimetres (Fig. 14.8), whereas in the most severe type the innominate bone, including the acetabulum, is shattered and driven inwards together with the femoral head (Fig. 14.9).

Diagnosis

The extent of the damage to the bone of the acetabulum may be difficult to assess from conventional radiography. The decision on which fractures of the acetabulum are suitable for surgical treatment has been simplified by the advent of more sophisticated imaging using computed tomographic (CT) scanning (Fig. 14.10). The technique is far superior to conventional anterior and posterior oblique plain radiographs, though these still have an important place in planning the most appropriate surgical approach.

Treatment

Severe shock may demand energetic resuscitation, and the possibility of major internal bleeding should be borne in mind.

Treatment of the skeletal injury depends largely upon the degree of comminution and displacement of the acetabular fragments, and upon whether or not it is possible to restore the articular surface to its normal shape. In practice the cases thus fall into two groups: (1) those in which the main part of the weight-bearing surface of the acetabulum can be restored to its normal position, congruous with the femoral head; and (2) those in which this is impossible on account of severe comminution of the weight-bearing surface.

Where restoration of the articular surface is possible, non-surgical treatment by skeletal traction through a femoral Steinmann pin will sometimes pull down the displaced fragment of the acetabulum, which should then remain congruent with the femoral head when traction is removed. Traction should, however, be maintained for 4–6 weeks until bony stability has developed. Surgical treatment is indicated when an anterior or posterior fracture–

Fig. 14.9 Severe central fracture–dislocation of the hip (arrows). There is no possibility of restoring a smooth acetabular surface.

Fig. 14.10 CT scans in two planes to show displaced fragments in severe central fracture–dislocation of the hip.

dislocation (Fig. 14.9) cannot be reduced by traction. Traction may be continued for symptomatic relief for 2 or 3 days while the fracture is fully evaluated and the most appropriate surgical treatment planned. Ideally, patients with these difficult fractures should be transferred to a unit that specialises in their treatment, but this should not be delayed for more than 7–10 days. The incision chosen for treatment depends on the location of the fracture and may require an anterior ilio-inguinal approach, an extended ilio-femoral approach, or sometimes a combined anterior and posterior approach. Following open reduction, fixation of the fragments may be achieved by a combination of multiple screws and contoured plates. In many instances it is necessary to use additional bone grafts to reconstitute skeletal defects resulting from fracture impaction. Surgical complications are frequent, particularly infection and thrombo-embolism and appropriate prophylactic treatment is required. Following surgery, light traction should be continued until wound healing has occurred and weight-bearing is deferred for at least 6 weeks.

The group in which severe comminution precludes accurate reduction presents major difficulties in management (Fig 14.9). Opinion is divided on whether to restrict active intervention to an attempt to draw the upper end of the femur and the shattered acetabulum out to somewhere near the anatomical position, or to adopt a more aggressive policy and by open operation to restore the fragments as accurately as possible to form a reasonably smooth socket congruous with the femoral head. In all these cases it is certainly worth accomplishing what one can by combined lateral and downward traction through pins transfixing the trochanter and the lower end of the femur.

It should be borne in mind that many patients with central dislocation of the hip will eventually need total replacement arthroplasty on account of secondary degenerative changes, and one of the objectives of the primary treatment should be to restore the hip sufficiently closely to its normal position to ensure that conditions are favourable for arthroplasty, should it be required.

Complications
As in other fractures of the pelvis (see p. 215) there may be severe haemorrhage from damage to a major blood vessel, but the common complication is degenerative arthritis from damage to the articular surface of the acetabulum. This may develop early (within a few months) or after a period of years. If the disability from arthritis becomes severe the only effective treatment is by operation. The choice usually lies between arthrodesis and total replacement arthroplasty.

FRACTURES OF THE PROXIMAL FEMUR

Classification

Fractures of the proximal femur, often described as fractures of the hip, are included in this chapter for convenience. They are classified as follows:

[1] Fracture of the neck of the femur
[2] Fracture of the trochanteric region

Fig. 14.11 Typical displaced fracture of the neck of the femur in Ⓐ antero-posterior and Ⓑ lateral view.

FRACTURE OF THE NECK OF THE FEMUR

Fracture of the neck of the femur is common in persons over the age of 60 years and is one of the so-called 'fatigue' fractures (see Chapter 1). Women are especially at risk, because of a tendency for their bone to become increasingly fragile after the menopause in consequence of generalised osteoporosis. The increasing incidence of these fractures in the ageing population has made them one of the commonest causes of morbidity, use of hospital care, and death in patients over the age of 65. The average mortality rate following fracture approaches 10% at 30 days post injury and reaches 30% after 1 year. These high mortality rates are often associated with comorbidities from chronic disease in other systems, particularly cardiovascular and respiratory disorders. Many patients will require specialised medical care to investigate and treat these disorders to enable them to undergo surgical treatment of the fracture itself. Wherever possible surgery should be performed within 24–48 hours from admission as further delay increases the incidence of life-threatening compli-cations in these already compromised patients.

The causative injury is often slight-usually a fall or stumble. In most cases the fracture is probably caused by a rotational force. In about 95% of cases, there is marked displacement, the shaft fragment being rotated laterally and displaced upwards, often with comminution of the posterior cortex (Fig. 14.11). In the remaining cases the two fragments are firmly impacted together, with slight abduction of the distal fragment upon the proximal (impacted abduction fracture, see Fig. 14.14).

Clinical features

Displaced fracture. A typical history is that the patient—usually an elderly woman—tripped and fell, and was unable to get up again unaided. She was subsequently unable to take weight on the injured limb. On examination the most striking feature is the marked lateral rotation of the limb. This is often as much as 90°, so that the patella and the foot point laterally. The limb is shortened by about 2–3 cm. Any movement of the hip causes severe pain.

Impacted abduction fracture (see Fig. 14.14). In the exceptional case in which the fracture is impacted, the history and signs are different. The patient may have been able to pick herself up after falling, and she may even have walked a few steps afterwards, perhaps with assistance. Indeed, some patients have remained mobile despite pain, and have not sought medical advice immediately. On examination there is no detectable shortening and no rotational deformity. The patient is able to move the hip through a moderate range without severe pain.

Radiographic examination. In the ordinary case with displacement of the fragments the fracture is obvious and cannot be mistaken (Fig. 14.11A), but in some cases of impacted abduction fracture the radiographic changes are slight and the fracture may be overlooked (see Fig. 14.14). Lateral radiographs should always be obtained, as well as antero-posterior films. Occasionally, in cases of doubt, it may be necessary to request an MRI or isotope bone scan to confirm the diagnosis.

Treatment

Displaced fractures and impacted abduction fractures must be considered separately.

Displaced fractures. A displaced fracture of the neck of the femur is one of the few fractures that needs rigid immobilisation if it is to have any chance of uniting. The alternative treatment, in which the femoral head is excised and replaced by a metal prosthesis, is more commonly used, especially when there is comminution of either fragment, severe displacement, and when the patient is elderly or debilitated.

Standard method of fracture fixation. For many years the device most commonly used for fracture fixation was the three-flanged Smith–Petersen nail or one of its modifications. Most surgeons now prefer to use a compression screw-plate (dynamic hip screw), or three parallel cannulated screws. A compression screw plate consists of a substantial coarse-threaded screw, the shank of which slides telescopically in a cylindrical barrel, prolonged distally into a plate which is screwed to the femoral shaft (Figs 14.12 & 14.13).

Prior to insertion of the fixation device the fracture is reduced on an orthopaedic table by manipulation and the patient checked by conventional radiography or image intensifier. When an acceptable position is achieved a small lateral incision is made over the base of the greater trochanter to allow trial guide wires to be passed up through the femoral neck into the head. The most suitable wire in both the antero-posterior and lateral view is selected and the length of fixation device required is then measured. If three cannulated screws are used, they can be inserted directly over parallel wires and screwed into the

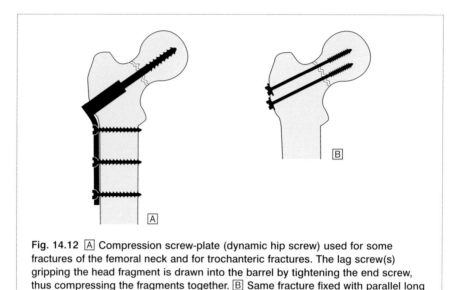

Fig. 14.12 [A] Compression screw-plate (dynamic hip screw) used for some fractures of the femoral neck and for trochanteric fractures. The lag screw(s) gripping the head fragment is drawn into the barrel by tightening the end screw, thus compressing the fragments together. [B] Same fracture fixed with parallel long screws.

Fig. 14.13 [A] Displaced fracture of neck of femur before reduction. [B] After manipulative reduction and fixation by a sliding screw-plate (dynamic hip screw).

femoral head to secure fixation. Insertion of the larger compression screw requires the preparation of a track using a special cannulated combined drill and tap. The coarse-threaded screw is then inserted into the femoral head with an introducer. The barrel of the device is then inserted over the screw and the plate section secured to the femoral shaft with cortical bone screws. If necessary,

Fig. 14.14 Impacted abduction fracture of the neck of the femur. Note that the shaft fragment is slightly abducted in relation to the femoral head, so that the upper corner of the fracture surface is driven into the cancellous bone of the femoral head. This is the only type of femoral neck fracture in adults that can be treated successfully without operation.

a tightening device in the barrel can be used to draw the screw gripping the femoral head back into the barrel, thus increasing compression and stability at the fracture site.

After operation the patient is nursed free in bed and active hip movements are encouraged. Most surgeons encourage early walking with the aid of crutches or a frame—within the first week after the operation—on the grounds that in these elderly patients the advantages to the general health of being up and about far outweigh the theoretical advantages to the fracture of rest.

Alternative methods for selected fractures in the elderly. Because of the uncertain results of fixing these fractures by internal devices, especially in the elderly, most surgeons now advise immediate excision of the femoral head and its replacement by a metal prosthesis (replacement arthroplasty, see Fig. 14.17A). Some go even further and advise total replacement arthroplasty, requiring the fitting of a plastic socket as well as a prosthetic femoral head (see Fig. 14.17B), if the bones are very soft. These operations are a little more severe than that of introducing parallel screws or a compression screw-plate, and they carry a higher mortality and complication rate. Despite this, the results are sufficiently encouraging to suggest that they merit a place in primary treatment, especially in elderly persons who recover their mobility more rapidly. It is accordingly common practice now at many centres to recommend primary prosthetic replacement or total replacement arthroplasty as a routine method in preference to internal fixation in patients over the age of 70.

Treatment in children. Femoral neck fracture is uncommon in children, but when it occurs most surgeons advise operative fixation, usually by two or three threaded pins, because bone healing is more reliable and complications fewer.

Impacted abduction fractures. It must be emphasised that a diagnosis of impacted abduction fracture should not be made unless both the clinical and radiological criteria of impaction are satisfied (Fig. 14.14). In the absence of such strict criteria, firm impaction of the fracture cannot be assumed, and there is a serious risk that the fragments will fall apart. Despite the feasibility of

Fig. 14.15 Normal blood supply of the femoral head. The three groups of vessels are: (1) vessels in ligament of femoral head; (2) capsular vessels; (3) nutrient vessels from the femoral shaft. A fracture through the femoral neck may leave only the vessels in the ligament of the femoral head intact, but some of the capsular vessels may also escape.

conservative treatment, there is an increasing trend towards routine internal fixation of impacted abduction fractures, because of a fear that displacement may occur.

Complications

Fractures of the neck of the femur are more prone to serious complications than is any other fracture. The important complications are avascular necrosis, non-union, and late osteoarthritis. All these complications affect fractures with displacement rather than impacted abduction fractures.

Avascular necrosis. After fracture of the femoral neck the blood supply to the head of the femur is precarious. Normally, blood is supplied to the femoral head by three routes (Fig. 14.15): through the vessels in the ligament of the head of the femur (ligamentum teres), through the capsular vessels reflected onto the femoral neck, and through branches of the nutrient vessels within the substance of the bone. When the neck of the femur is fractured the nutrient vessels within the bone are necessarily severed. Some at least of the capsular vessels are also likely to be interrupted, and the higher the fracture the more complete is the interruption of these channels likely to be. Thus the viability of the femoral head may depend almost entirely upon the blood supplied through the ligament of the head of the femur (ligamentum teres). This is a variable quantity, and it is often insufficient to keep the head alive. In that event the bone cells die (avascular necrosis) and the fracture may fail to unite, or if it does unite it may not do so quickly enough to allow revascularisation of the head fragment before irreversible changes in bone or cartilage have occurred. Depending upon the degree of ischaemia, avascular changes may be total, affecting the whole of the head, or they may be partial, affecting only a segment of the head.

Consequences. The main consequence of avascular necrosis of the head of the femur is collapse of the bone structure, leading to fragmentation (Fig. 14.20). This does not occur immediately but is delayed for months or even for as long as a year or more. Necrosis and collapse involving the fracture surface may lead to failure of union of the fracture, whereas collapse at the articular surface leads to degenerative arthritis (osteoarthritis). If necrosis is total the whole femoral head may collapse, with complete disorganisation of the hip. The complication of avascular necrosis is thus closely related to both of the other two complications to be described: non-union and osteoarthritis.

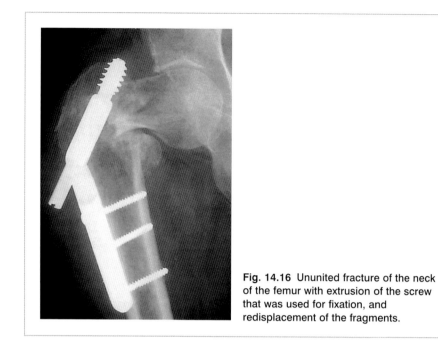

Fig. 14.16 Ununited fracture of the neck of the femur with extrusion of the screw that was used for fixation, and redisplacement of the fragments.

Treatment. Treatment is mainly that of the secondary effects and will be described in the succeeding sections on non-union and osteoarthritis.

Non-union. Non-union occurs in about a quarter to a third of all cases of fracture of the neck of the femur treated by internal fixation despite competent primary treatment. Three possible causes of non-union have to be considered: avascular necrosis, loss of fixation, and entry of synovial fluid from the joint into the fracture haematoma. A loss of the blood supply to the head fragment is probably the most important, as it will inhibit healing across the fracture site. Loss of implant fixation in the soft osteoporotic bone may result in increased mobility at the fracture site and also inhibits healing. The role of synovial fluid in preventing normal fracture haematoma formation is less certain, that is a factor that requires further investigation.

Pathology and clinical features. When the fracture fails to unite, the neck of the femur undergoes progressive absorption, so that the femoral head sinks down towards the trochanters. At the same time the fixation device loosens and loses its grip in the femoral head. Finally the screw or nail breaks away from the femoral head and the fragments become redisplaced (Fig. 14.16). As noted already, if the bone is avascular there may also be total or partial collapse of the femoral head, though this may be delayed for many months or even for 2 years or more.

Clinically, after seeming to make good progress at first, the patient begins to complain of renewed pain. Often there is sudden deterioration with acute pain, lateral rotation of the limb, shortening, and inability to walk, denoting breaking out of the fixation device. This disaster may take place at any time from a few weeks to 3 years from the time of the initial operation: it commonly occurs at 2–6 months.

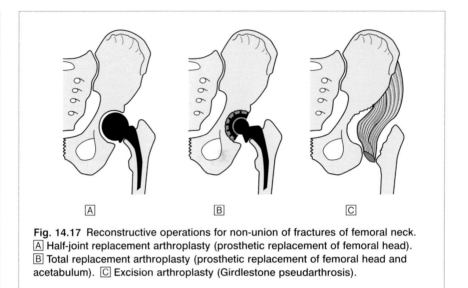

Fig. 14.17 Reconstructive operations for non-union of fractures of femoral neck. Ⓐ Half-joint replacement arthroplasty (prosthetic replacement of femoral head). Ⓑ Total replacement arthroplasty (prosthetic replacement of femoral head and acetabulum). Ⓒ Excision arthroplasty (Girdlestone pseudarthrosis).

Treatment. Non-union almost inevitably necessitates further operation, and this is especially true if it is associated with avascular necrosis and collapse of the femoral head. At the present time the choice of treatment generally lies in one of the following methods:

- simple removal of the fixation device without further treatment
- prosthetic replacement of femoral head (half-joint replacement arthroplasty, Fig. 14.17A)
- prosthetic replacement of femoral head with an articulating acetabular cup (biarticular arthroplasty)
- prosthetic replacement of femoral head and acetabulum (total replacement arthroplasty, Fig. 14.17B)
- excision arthroplasty (Fig. 14.17C).

In general, there is a strong preponderance of opinion in favour of replacement arthroplasty, either by prosthetic replacement of the femoral head alone or by total replacement arthroplasty.

Removal of the fixation device eliminates any local symptoms from prominence of the metal device in the thigh, but it has little effect in improving function. Nevertheless, some patients manage to get about to a limited extent without further treatment and, in patients who are elderly, frail and perhaps in consequence confined to one or two rooms, there may be no indication for more drastic measures.

Half-joint replacement arthroplasty (hemiarthroplasty), i.e. prosthetic replacement of the femoral head with a stemmed metal component, has for years been the mainstay of treatment for non-union of fractures of the neck of the femur and for collapse of the head from avascular necrosis, and it is still used widely for these conditions, though to some extent it has been superseded by bipolar (biarticular) arthroplasty or total replacement arthroplasty (see below). The operation consists in removal of the head and neck of the femur and replacement by a metal prosthesis, the stem of which enters the medullary canal of the femoral shaft (Figs 14.17A, 14.18 & 14.19), where it is usually

Fig. 14.18 [A] Femoral head prosthesis (Thompson pattern). [B] Radiograph after half-joint replacement arthroplasty for a femoral neck fracture. Acrylic cement, used to stabilise the prosthesis in the femur, is seen round the stem of the prosthesis. (The cement had been made radio-opaque by the addition of barium salts.)

embedded securely in acrylic filling compound or 'cement'. Walking with crutches is begun within a few days after the operation.

Bipolar (biarticular) replacement arthroplasty is a refinement of half-joint replacement arthroplasty. The artificial femoral head is enclosed within a loosely fitting plastic-lined cup, so that in effect there is a double articulation (biarticular cup) (Fig. 14.19): the aim of this refinement is to reduce wear of the acetabulum by pressure against it of an unyielding metal head. Whether or not this device will prove superior to a plain metal femoral head prosthesis is still uncertain.

Total replacement arthroplasty—that is, insertion of an artificial socket and a femoral head prosthesis (Fig. 14.17B)—is preferred to replacement of the femoral head alone in late cases with disorganisation of the acetabulum as well as of the femoral head. Indeed, many surgeons prefer to undertake this more radical operation even when the acetabulum appears healthy, on the grounds that it offers more certain relief of pain. It also forestalls an important complication sometimes seen after replacement of the femoral head alone—namely, erosion of the acetabulum with consequent upward and medial migration of the prosthetic femoral head, which may necessitate secondary total replacement arthroplasty.

In the case of excision arthroplasty (Girdlestone pseudarthrosis) the head and neck of the femur are excised and the side wall of the pelvis is smoothed by removing the upper margin of the acetabulum (Fig. 14.17C). A flap of muscle or other soft tissue (the gluteus medius muscle is appropriate) may be interposed as a cushion between the shaft of the femur and the pelvis. The

A

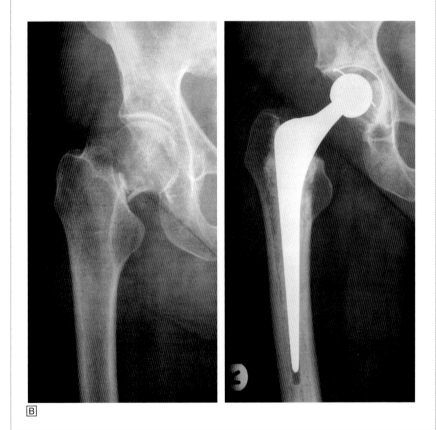

Fig. 14.19 [A] Replacement of the femoral head by a biarticular prosthesis for fracture of the femoral neck in an elderly patient. The femoral component moves within the cup while the cup is also free to move in the acetabulum. [B] Primary total hip replacement for severely displaced femoral neck fracture.

B

Fig. 14.20 Avascular necrosis of a large segment of the femoral head 2 years after fracture of the femoral neck. Although the fracture appears to have united, the ischaemic changes adjacent to the joint margin, with considerable collapse of the bone, are causing osteoarthritis.

effect is to create a false joint which is painless and has a reasonable range of movement, but with some shortening and instability. This method is seldom used as a first-choice operation, but it is useful as a salvage operation when deep infection has developed as a complication of internal fixation or hemiarthroplasty.

Osteoarthritis. Even when a fracture of the neck of the femur unites by bone there is a risk of the later development of osteoarthritis. Arthritis may arise (1) from mechanical damage to the articular cartilage at the time of injury or operation; (2) from impairment of the blood supply to the basal layers of the cartilage, which are probably nourished largely from the vessels in the underlying bone (Fig. 14.20); or (3) from union in faulty alignment. It may develop within months of the original injury, as is usually the case after avascular necrosis of the femoral head, or the onset may be delayed for as long as 20 years or more, as in cases of malalignment. Treatment is along the usual lines for osteoarthritis from other causes.

FRACTURE OF THE TROCHANTERIC REGION

The term trochanteric fracture[1] may be used to describe any fracture in the region that lies approximately between the greater and the lesser trochanter. It is unnecessary to retain such terms as 'intertrochanteric' and 'pertrochanteric', which only lead to confusion.

---

[1] It must be made clear that some surgeons use the term 'fracture of the neck of the femur' loosely to include trochanteric fractures as well as fractures of the femoral neck proper. Thus they recognise two types of femoral neck fracture: (1) intracapsular or transcervical fracture (= fracture of femoral neck proper), and (2) extracapsular or trochanteric fracture. Less confusion will arise if the classification suggested on page 223 is adopted.

Fig. 14.21 A typical trochanteric fracture before A and after B internal fixation with a compression screw-plate (dynamic hip screw).

A trochanteric fracture is a much more benign injury than a fracture of the neck of the femur, because it usually unites readily no matter how it is treated, and it is almost immune from the serious complications of avascular necrosis and non-union for which femoral neck fractures are notorious.

Trochanteric fractures are common in the elderly—especially in women, who form the bulk of the aged population. If anything, they have a higher average age incidence than femoral neck fractures. Thus they are seen very often in persons of 75–85 years. The cause is nearly always a fall superimposed on an underlying degree of osteoporosis. The injury forms one of the group of fatigue fractures (Chapter 6) and patients require investigation and treatment for the underlying bone loss.

Clinical features

The history is much the same as that in cases of fracture of the neck of the femur. After being knocked down or falling, the patient is unable to get up without assistance, and is unable to put weight on the limb. On examination the findings resemble those of a femoral neck fracture in that the limb is shortened and rotated laterally. Pain is most marked over the trochanteric region, and after a day or two a visible ecchymosis often appears at the back of the upper thigh—a feature not seen in cases of femoral neck fracture because extravasated blood is retained within the joint capsule.

Radiographic examination. In most cases the fracture is obvious (Fig. 14.21A), but a fracture without displacement may easily be overlooked. Careful scrutiny of good antero-posterior and lateral radiographs is required to determine whether there are two, three, or four fracture fragments (Fig. 14.22).

Fig. 14.22 Comminuted 4-part trochanteric fracture.

Treatment

Because trochanteric fractures unite readily, the main objects of treatment are to ensure that the fragments are held in good position and to encourage the patient in regaining perfect function. Early internal fixation is the treatment of choice in these older patients who are prone to develop life-threatening complications if subjected to prolonged rest in bed.

Standard method. Internal fixation by a compression screw-plate (dynamic hip screw) (Fig. 14.21B) is now the routine method of treatment. Its advantage is that for the more comminuted unstable fractures the sliding screw retains its fixation in the head despite some shortening at the fracture site.

After operation the patient is nursed free in bed, active hip and knee exercises being practised from the beginning. Usually, walking with the partial support of a walking frame or crutches is begun within 1 or 2 days of the operation. Early walking is especially important in the elderly because they tolerate inactivity badly. The technique of inserting a compression screw plate was described on page 225.

Alternative methods. A new type of two-component fixation device has been developed for the treatment of the more unstable oblique and comminuted sub-trochanteric fractures of the femur. These devices, such as the gamma nail, combine a short intramedullary nail with a nail or coarse-thread screw inserted within the femoral neck (Fig. 14.23). This configuration provides much more stable fixation for the fracture and allows early weight-bearing.

Complications

Trochanteric fractures have fewer major complications than fractures of the neck of the femur, but still develop significant problems of fixation failure, with non-union or mal-union occurring in 10–15% of unstable comminuted fractures.

Fig. 14.23 [A] Comminuted trochanteric fracture with sub-trochanteric extension.
[B] Trochanteric fracture after fixation with Gamma nail.

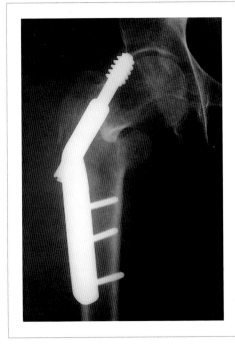

Fig. 14.24 Failure of fixation in a comminuted trochanteric fracture. The screw has cut out from the femoral head.

Failure of the fixation device. In severe comminuted trochanteric fractures, especially in patients with osteoporosis, there is an unpredictable incidence of early failure of the fixation device. Thus, if the bone is very soft it is not uncommon for the fixation screw to cut out from the femoral head (Fig. 14.24).

Mal-union. The only complication that is frequent is mal-union, and this is seldom severe. Despite the greatest care in treatment, many trochanteric fractures unite with a slightly reduced neck-shaft angle (coxa vara). This may occur through bending or breakage of a nail-plate, or simply through compression of the soft cancellous bone in contact with the metal. Coxa vara is associated with shortening, but this seldom exceeds 2 or 3 cm.

In neglected or untreated cases mal-union may be more troublesome, because the fracture may unite with marked lateral rotation of the shaft fragment as well as with severe coxa vara.

Treatment. In most cases mal-union can be accepted without treatment other than perhaps building up the shoe on the affected side to compensate for shortening. Occasionally a severe deformity may demand correction, especially if it occurs in a young person. The bone is divided in the trochanteric region and the fragments are secured in the correct position by a compression screw-plate or other appropriate device, as in the treatment of a fresh fracture.

15 | Thigh and knee

FRACTURES OF THE FEMUR
[1] Fracture of the neck of the femur, and

[2] Fracture of the trochanteric region (these fractures are dealt with in Chapter 14 but their anatomical position is included here for convenience)

[3] Fracture of the shaft of the femur
[4] Supracondylar fracture
[5] Condylar fracture

INJURIES OF THE KNEE
Fractures of the patella
Injuries of the extensor mechanism
Dislocation of the knee joint
Dislocation of the patella
Injuries of the ligaments of the knee
Tears of the menisci of the knee
Traumatic effusions in the knee

FRACTURE OF THE SHAFT OF THE FEMUR

Fracture of the shaft of the femur occurs at any age, usually from severe violence such as may be caused by a road accident or aeroplane crash. It may occur at any site, and is almost equally common in the uppermost, middle and lowest thirds of the shaft. Likewise the pattern of the fracture is variable, and may be transverse, oblique, spiral, comminuted (Fig. 15.1), or (in children) of the greenstick type. More often than not there is marked displacement of the fragments, in the form of angulation and overlap, and muscle may be interposed between the fragments. The fracture commonly results in a significant blood loss of 0.5–1.5 litres into the soft tissues of the thigh, which can result in hypovolaemic shock necessitating blood or fluid replacement.

The femur is a common site for pathological fractures from carcinomatous metastases. Fractures from this cause generally occur in the upper half of the bone (Fig. 15.2).

Radiographic examination. Radiographs should always include the hip and knee. A recognised error is to overlook a dislocation of the hip coexisting with a fracture of the femoral shaft.

Treatment

The well-tried method of conservative treatment by sustained weight traction with the limb supported in a Thomas's type splint has now been largely replaced by intramedullary nailing with interlocking screws as the method of

Fig. 15.1 Comminuted fracture of the shaft of the femur.

Fig. 15.2 A Pathological fracture of the femur from carcinomatous metastasis. This is a common site. B The same fracture after internal fixation with a long intramedullary nail with two proximal neck screws.

choice in the adult patient (see Fig. 15.6). With conservative treatment the period of disability is usually lengthy, though the results are nearly always excellent. The indications for internal fixation by a long intramedullary nail have widened in recent years with modern refinements in the technique of 'closed' nailing with image intensifier radiographic control and locking screws, proximally and distally. Nevertheless, it must be remembered that by no means every fracture of the femoral shaft lends itself well to intramedullary nailing: many comminuted fractures and fractures close to the upper or lower end are unsuitable. When nailing is done by the open method, with wide exposure of the fracture site—the method sometimes used—the complications of infection and of knee stiffness are more frequent.

Conservative treatment by traction and splintage. The principles of this method are to reduce the fracture by traction and manipulation, to support the limb in a Thomas's splint (p. 39) and to maintain continuous traction by the application of a suitable weight to preserve length until healing occurs.

An anaesthetic is not always required for reduction. Traction is applied to the lower leg, either by adhesive skin strapping, or by a Steinmann pin through the upper end of the tibia (see Fig. 15.3). A Thomas's splint with Pearson knee flexion attachment (Fig. 3.10, p. 38) or a similar splint is fitted. By a combination of traction and manipulation, under radiographic or image intensifier control, an attempt is made to bring the fragments into correct apposition and align-

Fig. 15.3 Model showing the correct site for transfixation of the tibia by a Steinmann pin for purposes of traction. The stirrup slips over the ends of the pin. Sometimes a length of piano wire (Kirschner wire) held taut between the limbs of a 'horse shoe' is used instead of the rigid steel pin.

ment. When satisfactory reduction has been achieved, the splintage and traction are adjusted to maintain the position. Canvas strips are slung between the bars of the Thomas's splint to support the thigh and calf with the knee flexed 15–20° to control rotation. The splint with the contained limb is suspended from an overhead beam by the balance-weight technique shown in Figure 15.4, and a suitable weight (4–6 kg, 10–15 lb, according to the build of the patient) is attached to the traction cord. Repeated check radiographs are advisable in the first 2 weeks, and appropriate adjustments to the slings or weights are made as required.

Rehabilitation. Exercises for the lower leg and foot are important in preserving muscle tone and in preventing deformity—especially that of equinus—and they should be begun immediately. As soon as the initial pain of the fracture begins to settle—usually about 1 week after the injury—active quadriceps and knee exercises are begun. Knee flexion through about 60° may be allowed, but more important than flexion is the ability to extend the knee fully by quadriceps action. These activities do not interfere with union of the fracture and may be encouraged with full confidence.

The duration of splintage varies from case to case. Except in children, few fractures of the femoral shaft are firmly joined in 12 weeks: most take 16 weeks or even longer. When the stage of sound union is reached the splint is removed and the patient is allowed to exercise freely in bed before walking is begun. Thereafter rehabilitation is continued until full function is restored.

Cast or functional bracing. In appropriate cases—usually those of fracture of the lower half of the femur and especially when the fracture is of the transverse or short oblique type—the period spent in bed with traction on the limb may be reduced by encasing the limb in a plaster spica or, preferably, in a plaster splint with hinged knee section (cast bracing; see p. 40). Once the fracture is becoming 'sticky'—usually 6–8 weeks after the injury—this functional brace may be substituted for the traction apparatus, and limited weight-bearing with the aid of crutches may be encouraged (Fig. 15.5). It is essential, however, to

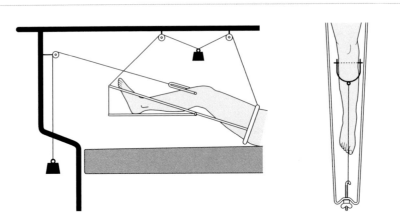

Fig. 15.4 Continuous traction with balanced suspension, using a Thomas's (or similar) splint with Pearson knee flexion attachment. This is the standard technique of traction for fractures of the shaft of the femur. The larger diagram shows the general layout of the cords and pulleys. The traction grip on the leg may be obtained by adhesive skin strapping or by a pin through the tibia (as shown here and in Fig. 15.4). There are two systems of cords and weights. The purpose of one system is to support the splint and the contained limb from the overhead beam. This weight is adjusted until the limb is nicely balanced. The purpose of the other system is to exert continuous traction in the line of the femur. Counter-traction is through the cords that suspend the splint from the beam, particularly the cord that is attached to the distal end of the splint; so it is unnecessary to raise the foot of the bed on blocks. Many modifications of this method of traction are in use but the basic principles are the same. One modification is shown in the smaller diagram: here a screw traction device attached to the end of the splint is used instead of the traction weight. This technique is termed 'fixed traction' as distinct from the 'sliding traction' shown in the larger diagram.

Fig. 15.5 Functional brace with plastic knee hinges used in the later stages of treatment of a mid-shaft fracture of the femur.

keep a close check on the alignment of the fragments, because in adverse circumstances—for instance if the cast-brace is applied imperfectly or too early, or if the thigh is obese—angulation at the fracture may occur and lead to mal-union.

Treatment by external fixation. External fixation entails penetration or transfixion of each fragment by stout threaded pins which are left protruding through the skin, and rigid anchorage of the pins to an external steel bar by clamps or by cement (see p. 41). The bone fragments are thus held rigidly in the reduced position. The method is applicable mainly to open fractures with contamination or to infected fractures, in which internal fixation may be unduly hazardous. External fixation offers the advantage that any wound is easily accessible for treatment.

Operative treatment with internal fixation. Internal fixation, usually by a long intramedullary nail, is now the accepted treatment of choice for the majority of adult femoral shaft fractures. The advantages of early mobilisation, with the reduction in the incidence of muscle wasting and joint stiffness, outweigh the slight risk of infection complicating the operation. Where suitable facilities are not available, or when the patient is unsuitable for surgery, conservative treatment in traction may be used. However, in the following circumstances facilities for operative fixation should be sought, if at all possible:

- When satisfactory reduction cannot be secured and maintained by manipulation and traction—as, for instance, when a large mass of muscle has become wedged between the fragments.
- In elderly frail persons who would be likely to respond unfavourably to a long period of rest in bed with relative immobility.
- In cases of severe multiple injuries to the lower limbs, to facilitate the management of the other injuries.
- In patients with pathological fractures, especially those from metastatic deposits (Fig. 15.6), to facilitate nursing and allow some restoration of function even if the fracture fails to unite.

Technique of intramedullary nailing for a femoral fracture. Whenever possible, nailing should be done by the closed technique—that is, without exposing the fracture itself. The patient is placed in the lateral position, lying on the sound side, with the knee and lower leg of the affected side supported on a bridge or platform. To secure and maintain reduction of the fracture it may be necessary to apply strong traction upon the leg through a Steinmann pin inserted through the tibial tubercle or through the lower end of the femur. Through a lateral incision over the trochanteric region a long guide wire is introduced near the tip of the greater trochanter and passed down the shaft of the femur until its tip reaches the level of the fracture. The fragments are manipulated into correct apposition and alignment under radiographic control (preferably with an image-intensifier unit), whereupon the guide wire is passed on into the distal fragment of the femur, well into the condylar region. With special power-operated cannulated reamers the medullary canal is enlarged to the diameter of the nail that has been selected—usually about 12–16 mm. A nail of the correct length, and suitably curved to match the natural curve of the femoral shaft, is then threaded over the guide wire and driven home, the final position being checked again by radiographs.

Thigh and knee

Fig. 15.6 Severely displaced mid-shaft fracture of femur after fixation with intermedullary nail and interlocking screws.

When closed nailing is impracticable the open method may have to be used. The fracture is exposed through a small postero-lateral incision and the proximal fragment reamed in a retrograde direction. The selected nail is then inserted into the proximal fragment at the fracture site (Fig.15.7A) and driven backwards to protrude through the greater trochanter and allowed to emerge through a small incision in the skin of the buttock over its tip (Fig.15.7B). The fracture can then be accurately reduced under direct vision and the nail driven back down into the distal fragment to secure fixation (Fig.15.7C).

Locking screws. In recent years there has been an increasing trend towards locking the nail in place at the upper and lower ends by the insertion of cross-screws through holes provided at each end of the nail. The locking screws prevent rotation of the nail and thus increase stability.

Post-operative treatment. If it has been possible to secure rigid fixation with a strong nail of adequate diameter there is no need to immobilise the thigh in

Fig. 15.7 In open nailing of the femur the nail is first driven into the proximal fragment from the fracture site A and out through the greater trochanter B. After reduction of the fracture the nail is then engaged in the distal fragment C and driven home. (In practice a curved nail to match the natural curve of the femoral shaft is preferred to a straight nail.)

plaster or a splint. The patient may lie free in bed and practise exercises for the hip and knee joints and related muscles. Walking may be begun with the partial support of crutches 2 or 3 weeks after operation, or sometimes even sooner.

Treatment of femoral fractures in children

Treatment in young children: 'gallows' or Bryant's traction.[1] This method of traction is convenient and satisfactory for children up to the age of 3 years. By means of adhesive skin strapping applied direct to the skin of the legs, the child's lower limbs are suspended from an overhead beam. The cords are tightened just enough to raise the child's buttocks clear of the mattress (Fig. 15.8A). The weight of the pelvis and lower trunk is sufficient to maintain full length of the fractured femur, and the vertical position of the limb, together with the sustained suspension, automatically ensures good alignment. Small children tolerate this rather grotesque position without complaint. Since fractures

[1] Sir Thomas Bryant, a general surgeon working at Guy's Hospital, London, described this method of traction in 1873.

Thigh and knee

Fig. 15.8 [A] 'Gallows' or Bryant's traction for fractures of the femoral shaft in children of up to 3 years old. The cords are attached to an overhead beam. Note that the buttocks are suspended just clear of the mattress, so that the weight of the lower part of the trunk and pelvis exerts continuous traction on the limbs. The knees should be held slightly flexed by the simple plastic splint shown in [B], included beneath the crepe bandages.

unite rapidly in early childhood it is seldom necessary to maintain the suspension for more than 3 or 4 weeks.

Caution. In children suspended in 'gallows' traction the knees should be kept slightly flexed by simple back-splints (Fig. 15.8B) held in position with crepe bandages. Neglect of this precaution has led, very rarely, to spasm of the major artery of the limb and consequent ischaemia—a disastrous complication. It is also imperative that the strips of adhesive strapping used to support the limbs be applied direct to the skin, and not over encircling bandages: otherwise the limb may be constricted, with serious detriment to the circulation. As after all injuries to the limbs, the state of the circulation should be watched carefully, especially during the first 3 days.

In children older than 5 years, the prolonged bed rest required for conventional traction may be undesirable for both medical and social reasons. In these young patients alternative less invasive surgical techniques are now available that will facilitate early mobilisation. An external fixator can be applied to pins inserted into the femoral shaft above and below the fracture and will provide adequate stability while fracture healing occurs. The alternative is to use internal fixation with two flexible intramedullary pins inserted under image intensifier control through minimal incisions. These are much thinner than the conventional nails used in the adult and are inserted into the shaft through the metaphysis, thus avoiding damage to the epiphyseal growth plates.

Complications

The following complications of femoral shaft fractures will be considered:

Simultaneous dislocation of the hip. Radiographs should always include the hip lest a dislocation be overlooked, as has happened many times.

Injury to a major artery. Rarely, a sharp edge of the fractured bone may penetrate the soft tissues and damage the femoral artery. The vessel may be severed or it may be severely contused and occluded. In either case the outlook for the viability of the limb is grave unless continuity of the vessel can be restored by immediate operation.

Injury to a nerve. Just as a major artery may be damaged, so a nerve trunk may be struck by a sharp fragment of bone at the time of the initial injury. The severity of the damage can vary from transient neuropraxia to complete severance of the nerve. The sciatic nerve is obviously the most significant in this type of injury. As the nerve is broad and may divide into tibial and common peroneal components high up in the thigh, one or other of these subdivisions may be injured while the other escapes. The management of peripheral nerve injuries was discussed on page 64.

Infection. In cases of open (compound) fracture, contamination with consequent infection of the bone is an important potential complication. Clearly the risk of infection increases proportionately to the severity of the trauma and the degree of contamination. Thus in fractures that are 'compound from within', in which the skin is merely pierced from inside by a sharp fragment of bone, contamination may be negligible and the risk of osteomyelitis very slight. At the other extreme is the gunshot or bomb wound in which there is always heavy contamination and extensive tissue damage, and in these cases risk of infection is very high indeed.

Treatment is along the lines suggested on page 53. It must be re-emphasised here that in the management of a heavily contaminated wound such as a gunshot wound it is not permissible ever to close the wound by primary suture: such closure courts disaster. The correct treatment is to leave the wound open after initial cleansing and then, if the wound appears healthy and free from major infection, to undertake delayed primary suture after a few days.

Delayed union. Four months is a fair average time for union of a fractured femoral shaft in an adult. There is no hard-and-fast time limit beyond which union is said to be delayed, but if union is still insufficient to allow unprotected weight bearing after 5 months' support in a splint, additional methods of treatment must be considered.

Treatment. When callus is forming satisfactorily but is building up very slowly it is often wise to apply a cast-brace (p. 40) and to allow the patient to walk. This method will often obviate the need for operation, but it is appropriate to the young and active patient rather than to the elderly. In other cases some form of bone grafting operation may offer the best solution to the problem, as for non-union. If cross screws (locking screws) have been inserted at both ends of an intramedullary nail, removal of the screws at one or other end will often allow union to proceed.

Non-union. If union fails to occur and the fracture surfaces are becoming rounded and sclerotic, operation should be advised. The bone ends are freshened and bone grafts are applied. Internal fixation may be secured by a long intramedullary nail and the bone supplied in the form of slivers or chips of cancellous bone packed firmly about the site of fracture. If non-union proves unusually refractory and fails to respond to these measures there may be a place for treatment by electrical stimulation (p. 56).

Mal-union. Without constant supervision the fragments may suffer redisplacement in the form of angulation or overlap, and unless this is recognised the fracture will unite in the position of deformity. The most common examples of mal-union are overlap with consequent shortening, and lateral bowing. Lateral bowing is especially common when the fracture is in the upper half of the femur, and it has been seen more often since the over-enthusiastic adoption by some surgeons of early cast bracing for femoral fractures. An angular deformity may have secondary effects years later in the form of osteoarthritis of the knee (Fig. 4.14, p. 72).

Treatment. In most cases mal-union of slight or moderate degree is best accepted, the shoe being built up if necessary to correct shortening. It is a formidable undertaking to reproduce the fracture by osteotomy, realign the fragments and fix them with an intramedullary nail, but some such procedure may be advisable occasionally for mal-union of severe degree, especially if the patient is a young adult.

Stiffness of the knee. After a fracture of the femoral shaft the patient nearly always has some difficulty in regaining a full range of knee movement, but it is seldom that troublesome stiffness persists permanently. In most such cases stiffness is due not to a disturbance of the knee itself (because the joint is usually uninjured), but to periarticular and intramuscular adhesions which prevent free gliding of the muscle fibres one upon another, and to adhesions between the muscles and the femur.

Treatment. In most cases knee stiffness from a femoral shaft fracture responds well to treatment by active exercises if they are carried out intensively and for a long enough time. Many months may elapse before full recovery is gained. If the knee is uninjured and is therefore free from intra-articular adhesions, dramatic improvement cannot be expected from manipulation, and the temptation to force movement passively should be resisted.

In the rare cases in which knee stiffness is severe and is resistant to conscientious treatment by exercises, the range of movement may be increased by the operation of quadricepsplasty, in which all adhesions are divided and the quadriceps expansion may be freed further by division of its vastus medialis and vastus lateralis components. Quadricepsplasty demands prolonged and intensive after-treatment and is suitable only for robust adult patients. When adhesions within the joint are the main cause of stiffness, arthroscopic division of the adhesions is satisfactory.

SUPRACONDYLAR FRACTURE OF THE FEMUR

Although there is no strict line of demarcation between a low fracture of the femoral shaft and a supracondylar fracture, it is well to consider supracondylar fractures as a separate group because their treatment differs in certain respects from that of femoral shaft fractures.

Typically the fracture occurs just proximal to the point where the medial and lateral cortices of the femur flare out to form the condyles (Fig. 15.9). A vertical extension of the fracture may split the two condyles apart, giving a T-shaped

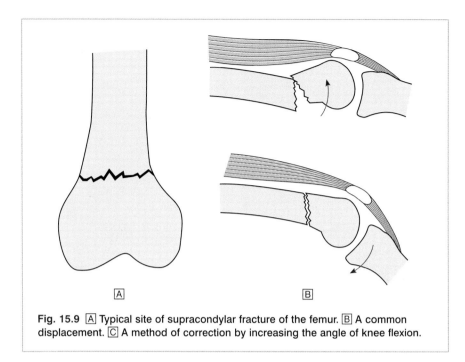

Fig. 15.9 Ⓐ Typical site of supracondylar fracture of the femur. Ⓑ A common displacement. Ⓒ A method of correction by increasing the angle of knee flexion.

fracture line, and sometimes there is more extensive comminution. Usually the main fracture is more or less transverse, and commonly the distal fragment is tilted anteriorly upon the shaft, without serious loss of end-to-end apposition (Fig. 15.9B).

Treatment

Although it is possible to treat supracondylar fractures of the femur con-servatively along the lines used for fractures of the femoral shaft, the tendency now is to rely in most cases upon operative fixation by a condylar screw-plate or nail plate.

Non-operative management. Most supracondylar fractures of the femur may be treated successfully by supporting the limb on a Thomas's splint with a knee flexion attachment, with continuous weight traction, as for fractures of the femoral shaft (see Fig. 15.4). But whereas in fractures of the femoral shaft the position of the knee is unimportant and is dictated mainly by considerations of comfort and convenience, in displaced supracondylar fractures the angle of knee flexion is often the key to the problem of reduction and stabilisation of the fracture. This point is illustrated in Figures 15.9B and C, where it is seen that forward tilting of the distal fragment may be corrected by increasing the angle of knee flexion. The appropriate position for the knee is determined in the light of successive radiographs obtained during the first few days after the injury.

In supracondylar fractures, unlike fractures of the femoral shaft proper, it is unwise to begin knee movements in the early days of treatment because the position of the fragments may be disturbed. For the first 2 or 3 weeks, physio-therapy for the injured limb should be restricted to active ankle, foot and toe exercises, and static contractions of the quadriceps and gluteal muscles. Knee

Fig. 15.10 Radiographs showing use of a condylar nail-plate for fixation of a supracondylar fracture of the femur.

movements should be begun as soon as the fracture has become stable, usually 2 or 3 weeks after the injury.

Cast-bracing. Supracondylar fractures of the femur are eminently suitable for treatment by cast or functional bracing (see p. 40) as soon as the fracture shows signs of commencing union-often about 4–6 weeks after the injury. The cast-brace allows walking with partial weight bearing, and the knee hinge incorporated in the brace permits the continuation of flexion and extension exercises.

Plaster spica. Supracondylar fractures without displacement may be treated by immobilising the limb in a plaster hip spica (or even in a long leg plaster if the patient is thin), and encouraging the patient to walk with sticks or crutches. This method is appropriate for children. The plaster may be changed for a functional brace at the appropriate time.

Operative reduction and internal fixation. Operative fixation has become the standard method of treatment and it is certainly the method of choice for elderly patients to avoid prolonged recumbency. The problems of operation are mainly technical: the distal fragment is short, often comminuted, and not well controlled by an intramedullary nail. The best fixation device is probably a combined (one-piece) nail-plate or a sliding screw and plate (dynamic condylar screw). The nail or screw is driven horizontally across the lower fragment and the plate, at right angles to the nail, is screwed to the outer side of the main upper fragment (Fig. 15.10).

Complications

Most supracondylar fractures unite readily: delayed union and non-union are infrequent. Otherwise the common complications are the same as those of fractures of the femoral shaft, namely mal-union and stiffness of the knee. Rarely, a badly displaced supracondylar fracture may be complicated by injury to the popliteal artery or to a major nerve trunk.

FRACTURES OF THE FEMORAL CONDYLES

Condylar fractures of the femur are uncommon injuries, usually caused by direct violence to the region of the knee. Two patterns of fracture are illustrated in Figure 15.11. The fracture may be no more than a crack without displacement, or there may be complete separation of a condyle with marked displacement.

Treatment

This depends upon the degree of displacement.

Undisplaced fractures may be treated by immobilisation in a long leg plaster (see Fig. 15.12) for about 6–8 weeks, walking being allowed from an early stage.

Displaced fractures demand accurate reduction because persistent displacement must inevitably disturb the mechanics of the knee and may lead to the later development of osteoarthritis. Reduction should first be attempted by traction and manipulation: if these are successful the limb is supported in a Thomas's splint with continuous weight traction, or in a full-length plaster.

If perfect reduction cannot be secured by traction and manipulation, operative reduction and internal fixation should be advised. The method of fixation to be used will depend upon the nature of the individual fracture: in most cases a separated condyle can best be held in position by multiple cancellous lag screws.

For a T-shaped fracture (Fig. 15.10) a right-angled compression screw-plate (dynamic condylar screw) is satisfactory. This grips and compresses the condylar fragments together, and the plate section is screwed to the outer side of the femoral shaft.

Complications

Stiffness of the knee. Most patients have difficulty in regaining a full range of knee movements. Stiffness is caused partly by intra-articular adhesions and partly by peri-articular and intramuscular adhesions. Treatment is mainly by active exercises. Gentle manipulation may be permissible later if steady progress is not being made with exercises alone. Resistant intra-articular adhesions may be divided arthroscopically.

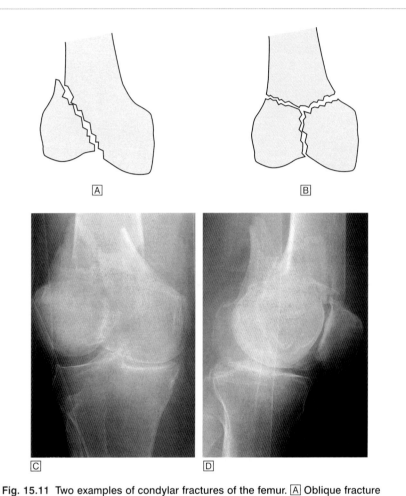

Fig. 15.11 Two examples of condylar fractures of the femur. [A] Oblique fracture shearing the lateral condyle, which is here shown displaced upwards. [B]–[D] T-shaped fracture separating both condyles.

Osteoarthritis of the knee. Osteoarthritis may develop months or years after the injury if the joint surface is left roughened or if the femoral condyles are out of alignment; hence the importance of accurate reduction in the primary treatment of the fracture.

Injury to an artery or nerve. In violent injuries with marked displacement of a condylar fragment there may be direct mechanical injury to the popliteal artery or to one of the main nerve trunks. These are rare complications, but it is important that they be recognised promptly. This emphasises again the necessity of looking routinely for signs of arterial or nerve injury at the first examination of every patient with a limb injury. The treatment of arterial injuries was described on page 62, and of nerve injuries on page 64.

Fig. 15.12 Postero-anterior radiograph of bipartite patella showing smaller unfused ossification centre (arrows).

INJURIES OF THE KNEE

FRACTURES OF THE PATELLA

Fractures of the patella may be caused by two types of injury: (1) a sudden violent contraction of the quadriceps muscle—as in attempting to preserve the balance after stumbling—and (2) a fall or blow directly on the knee cap. Muscular violence usually causes a clean break with separation of the fragments, whereas a direct blow causes a crack fracture or a comminuted fracture. Pain is severe and well localised, and haemarthrosis is to be expected.

Diagnosis

Radiographically the fracture is shown best by postero-anterior and lateral projections. Occasionally oblique or skyline views may be required to visualise small osteo-chondral fragments. The clinical and radiographic features usually make the diagnosis obvious, though occasionally a congenitally bipartite patella may be confused with a fracture. In this common anomaly the patella ossifies from two centres, instead of one, and the centres fail to coalesce. The smaller unfused centre commonly occupies the supero-lateral corner of the patella in postero-anterior radiographs (Fig. 15.12). It can be differentiated from a fracture fragment by the presence of smooth, non-jagged edges at the gap, which has sclerotic cortical margins on each side, and by the absence of any local tenderness.

Treatment

The treatment depends upon the type of fracture and, in some cases, upon the age of the patient. Three groups must be considered, as shown in Figure 15.13.

Fig. 15.13 Fractures of the patella and their treatment. The diagrams in the upper row show the three types of fracture, and those below depict the treatment for each type. A Crack without displacement. Treatment: Protection in walking plaster. B Clean break with separation of fragments. Treatment: Fix fragments with screw or excise patella. C Comminuted fracture with displacement. Treatment: Excise patella.

Crack fracture. In undisplaced crack fractures there is no fear of separation occurring later because the aponeurosis clothing the patella on its anterior and lateral aspects is intact and holds the fragments in position. Treatment is required only to relieve pain and to preserve and restore function. If there is a painfully tense haemarthrosis the blood should be aspirated. A plaster extending from groin to malleoli, with the knee in a position just short of full extension, should be worn for 3 weeks. Thereafter active exercises designed to redevelop the quadriceps muscle and to restore full mobility of the knee are practised under the supervision of a physiotherapist until full function is restored.

Clean break with separation of the fragments. Operation is required. Its nature should depend upon the quality of the bone and the extent of damage to the articular surface. Normally the fragments may be coapted accurately and fixed together rigidly by tension band wiring (Fig. 15.14), or with cannulated lag screws (Fig. 15.13). Reduction must be perfect and the fragments in intimate contact, as any residual irregularity in the articular surface will inevitably cause later osteoarthritis. Where accurate reduction is not possible because of

Fig. 15.14 Lateral radiograph showing tension band wiring for fixation of a fracture of the patella.

comminution at the fracture site in osteoporotic bone it is better to excise the patella.

After internal fixation of a fractured patella the knee should be protected in plaster for 2–3 weeks to allow healing of the soft tissues. If fixation is satisfactory it should then be possible to begin active knee flexion and quadriceps exercises under the supervision of a physiotherapist. Early walking with elbow crutches is encouraged, but unprotected weight-bearing should be avoided for 6 weeks.

Comminuted fracture. In comminuted fractures with displacement it is impossible to restore a perfectly smooth articular surface, so it is best to excise the patella. Only thus can the risk of troublesome osteoarthritis be avoided.

In excision of the patella the bone is dissected from the aponeurosis of the quadriceps, which closely invests it, and the aponeurosis is reconstructed by absorbable sutures, tension being relaxed by holding the knee fully extended. After operation the knee is protected in plaster in almost full extension for 3 weeks, in the latter half of which active quadriceps exercises and leg raising exercises are encouraged. After removal of the plaster, exercises are continued to restore movement and to redevelop the quadriceps muscle.

Results of excision of the patella. Excision of the patella gives excellent results provided the operation and the after-treatment are carried out efficiently. The function of the knee is not quite so perfect as that of the normal knee: the power of full extension is slightly impaired because the mechanical advantage that the patella affords by holding the tendon away from the axis of movement is lost. If any disability is noticed by these patients it is usually in climbing or descending ladders or stairs.

OTHER INJURIES OF THE EXTENSOR MECHANISM OF THE KNEE

In injuries from sudden muscular violence the quadriceps apparatus may give way at one of three points, as shown in Figure 15.15: (1) at the point of attachment of the quadriceps tendon to the upper pole of the patella; (2) through the patella and surrounding quadriceps expansion (fractured patella, see above) or (3) at the attachment of the patellar tendon to the tibial tubercle.

Avulsion from the patella. Avulsion of the quadriceps tendon from the upper pole of the patella occurs mainly in elderly men, in whom the tendon is often degenerate. The tendon should be reattached to the bone by sutures of stainless steel wire inserted through drill holes in the bone. Thereafter the knee should be protected by a full-length plaster for 6–8 weeks.

Avulsion at the tibial tubercle. This is the least common injury, occurring mainly in children or young adults. A fragment of bone may be pulled off with the tendon. This fragment should be fixed back to the tibia with a small screw and reinforced with a soft tissue repair.

DISLOCATION OF THE KNEE

Despite its rather flat articular surfaces, which do not afford intrinsic stability, the knee is dislocated less often than the other major joints: indeed, a dislocated knee must be regarded as a rare injury. This is fortunate, because dislocation of the knee is frequently complicated by injury to the popliteal artery or to one of the major nerve trunks.

Normally the knee is held stable by its strong ligaments (the two cruciate ligaments, the medial and lateral ligaments and the joint capsule) and by the protective control of the powerful quadriceps muscle. Dislocation is possible only if some or all of the ligaments are ruptured. The tibia may be displaced backwards, forwards, laterally or medially upon the femur.

Treatment

The dislocation should be reduced by traction and manipulation or, failing that, by operation. Thereafter the knee should be supported in a full-length lower

Fig. 15.15 The three points at which the quadriceps apparatus may rupture. (1) At insertion of quadriceps into patella; (2) through the patella; (3) at insertion of patellar tendon into tibial tubercle.

limb plaster (see Fig. 16.7) for 8–10 weeks before mobilising and muscle-strengthening exercises are begun.

Complications

The complications most to be feared are injuries of the popliteal artery and of the major nerve trunks behind the knee, all of which are especially vulnerable when the tibia is displaced backwards upon the femur. Arterial injury in particular demands urgent reconstructive surgery if the viability of the limb is not to be prejudiced. Less serious complications include persistent instability of the knee, restriction of knee movement and late osteoarthritis.

LATERAL DISLOCATION OF THE PATELLA

Lateral dislocation of the patella is recognised in three types: (1) acute dislocation, a single isolated injury; (2) recurrent dislocation and (3) habitual dislocation, in which the patella dislocates every time the knee is flexed. In recurrent dislocation and in habitual dislocation the knee shows abnormalities—often developmental-that render the patella unstable.

Acute dislocation

As a result of an injury while the knee is flexed or semi-flexed the patella is displaced laterally over the lateral femoral condyle and lies at the outer side of the knee. Clinically, the patient is unable to straighten the knee unless reduction occurs spontaneously or the patella is pushed back into position. Later the knee swells from an effusion of fluid, which may be bloodstained if the medial part of the capsule is torn. There is well-marked local tenderness antero-medially from strain or rupture of the capsule. The presence of a blood-stained effusion may also indicate the possibility of an osteochondral fracture from the articular surface of the patella. Post-reduction radiology, including skyline views, may be required to identify this common associated injury.

Treatment

The dislocation is easily reduced by applying medialward pressure upon the patella while the knee is gradually straightened. After a few days' rest with firm bandaging, a course of quadriceps exercises should be arranged. If an associated osteochondral fracture is present an arthroscopy will be required for its re-attachment or removal depending on its size.

Recurrent dislocation

Recurrent dislocation of the patella is seen most commonly in girls. The first dislocation generally occurs during adolescence. Thereafter, dislocations tend to recur with increasing ease, usually when the knee is being straightened from a flexed or semi-flexed position. The patient often shows generalised congenital joint laxity and may regard herself as 'double-jointed'. In addition, one or more of the following abnormalities may make the patella unstable: (1) a shallow intercondylar groove of the femur with underdeveloped lateral condyle; (2) a high-lying, rather small patella, which therefore rests in the shallow upper part of the intercondylar groove and (3) genu valgum, in consequence of which the line of pull of the quadriceps muscle is shifted further laterally than normal.

Treatment

If frequently recurring dislocations cause troublesome disability, operation should be advised. A reliable method is to detach the bony insertion of the patellar tendon and transpose it to a new bed in the tibia, medial and distal to the original insertion. In this way the patella is drawn lower into the intercondylar groove of the femur, and the line of pull of the quadriceps is transferred more to the medial side.

Because of the abnormal mechanics of the joint there is a risk that degenerative arthritis may develop in later life, even after a seemingly successful operation.

Habitual dislocation

Habitual dislocation is uncommon. It occurs at a much younger age than recurrent dislocation, often in early childhood. The underlying cause is shortening of the quadriceps muscle—particularly its vastus lateralis component—possibly from fibrosis following intramuscular injections in infancy. Sometimes there is an abnormal fibrous band tethering the vastus lateralis to the ilio-tibial tract. In consequence of the shortening or tethering of the muscle at the outer side, the patella is pulled laterally out of its groove every time the knee is flexed. In the absence of treatment the patella may eventually become permanently dislocated. Treatment is by releasing the tight muscle or band by dividing as much of it as is necessary to permit full flexion of the knee without displacement of the patella.

INJURIES OF THE LIGAMENTS OF THE KNEE

Injuries of the ligaments of the knee—common in athletes and sportsmen—often create serious problems and may lead to lasting disability. Whereas simple strains and partial ruptures heal well and allow full restoration of function—albeit often after a rather long interval—complete rupture of a ligament may cause permanent laxity with consequent instability of the knee.

In recent years surgeons have tended to adopt a more aggressive attitude to major tears of the knee ligaments, advising repair or reconstruction much more readily than was the case in the past, and the results probably justify this more active approach, even though in many cases the outcome is still imperfect.

Injuries of the ligaments of the knee may be classified into four groups:

1. Tear of the medial ligament (with or without the cruciate ligaments)
2. Tear of the lateral ligament (with or without the cruciate ligaments)
3. Tears of the cruciate ligaments alone
4. Strains or incomplete tears.

Tear of the medial ligament

This is caused by an injury that abducts the tibia upon the femur (Fig. 15.16A). The joint is momentarily subluxated, as shown in the diagram, but when the patient is seen, the subluxation has nearly always been reduced spontaneously. Wide abduction of the tibia upon the femur cannot occur unless the cruciate ligaments and the capsule are torn as well as the medial ligament (Fig. 15.16B). The medial meniscus may be torn at the same time, but it often escapes injury.

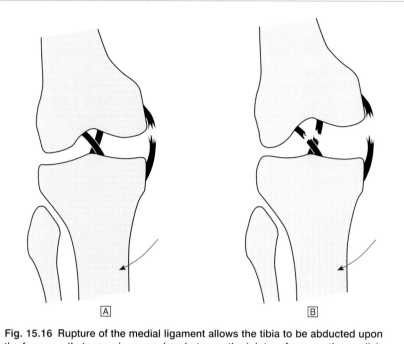

Fig. 15.16 Rupture of the medial ligament allows the tibia to be abducted upon the femur so that a gap is opened up between the joint surfaces on the medial side Ⓐ. If a wide gap is opened up it is almost certain that the capsule and one or both of the cruciate ligaments have been torn as well as the medial ligament Ⓑ.

Clinical features

The knee often contains blood-stained fluid. Effusion is not tense, however, because the fluid can escape from the joint cavity into the soft tissues through the rent. The point of greatest tenderness is along the course of the medial ligament, usually at its upper end, close to its attachment to the femur.

Diagnosis

Radiological determination of the integrity or otherwise of the ligament is conclusive. Antero-posterior radiographs are taken while an abduction stress is applied to the tibia, with the patient anaesthetised. If there is complete rupture of the ligament the joint will be shown to open up at the medial side (Fig. 15.16A). If the joint opens up widely (Fig. 15.16B) it is likely that the cruciate ligaments and capsule are torn as well as the medial ligament. The anterior draw test and the Lachman test indicate the integrity or otherwise of the cruciate ligaments, and the state of the ligaments and of the meniscus may be determined precisely by arthroscopy.

Treatment

Treatment may be non-operative or operative. Some surgeons prefer the one method, some the other; good results have been claimed for both. In relatively minor injuries with only slight abduction of the tibia upon the femur when examined under anaesthesia, conservative treatment is probably adequate, because the capsular rent is unlikely to be extensive or the ends of the ligament widely separated. For major tears involving the ligament and capsule, operation is now generally advised.

Conservative treatment. Aspiration may be required to remove a blood-stained effusion. The knee is then supported in a long-leg plaster, which may or may not include the foot, according to individual preference. The plaster is moulded closely about the limb to prevent abduction of the tibia on the femur. The patient is allowed to walk in the plaster, which is retained for 6 weeks. Thereafter, intensive exercises are carried out to mobilise the knee and to redevelop the quadriceps muscle.

Operative treatment. The knee is explored through a medial or antero-medial incision to determine the extent of the tear and to ascertain whether the medial meniscus and the cruciate ligaments are intact. If the meniscus is torn it should be removed, but if it is simply detached at the periphery the rent may be repaired by sutures. A torn cruciate ligament is generally best left alone in the acute stage (see below). Finally, the rent in the capsule and in the medial ligament itself is sutured. After operation the knee is supported in plaster for 6 weeks, and the subsequent treatment is the same as for patients treated without operation.

Tear of the lateral ligament

Tear of the lateral ligament is much less common than that of the medial. It is caused by a force adducting the tibia upon the femur. In some injuries of this type the ligament withstands the stress but the bony insertion of the ligament into the head of the fibula is avulsed with a fragment of bone. In other respects the injury is almost a mirror-image of a medial ligament tear, and the clinical features and treatment are comparable.

Complications
If the tibia is markedly adducted in relation to the femur at the time of injury—even though the displacement be momentary—there is a serious risk of injury to the common peroneal nerve from stretching. The effects of a severe stretch injury of the nerve are often irrecoverable.

Tears of the cruciate ligaments

The cruciate ligaments are sometimes torn with the medial or the lateral ligament, as has been mentioned already. Isolated tears of one or other of the cruciate ligaments may also occur. The anterior ligament is torn by a force driving the upper end of the tibia forwards relative to the femur, or by hyperextension of the knee. The posterior ligament is torn by a force driving the upper end of the tibia backwards.

Diagnosis
Normally, the anterior cruciate ligament prevents anterior glide of the tibia upon the femur, and the posterior cruciate ligament prevents posterior glide. Therefore in tears of the anterior cruciate ligament, when the knee is flexed 90° and the quadriceps muscle is relaxed the tibia can be drawn forwards

excessively compared with the normal side (anterior draw test). Instability may likewise be demonstrated by moving the upper end of the tibia forwards upon the femur with the knee flexed only 10 or 20° (Lachman test). In tears of the posterior cruciate ligament there is excessive posterior shift of the upper end of the tibia upon the femur when backward force is applied below the patella: even with the knee at rest the contour of the knee as seen from the side is altered, so that the upper end of the tibia is seen to sag backwards.

Treatment

Anterior cruciate tears. In tears of the anterior cruciate ligament the current trend is not to attempt immediate direct suture, which is technically unsatisfactory and often ineffective in restoring stability. Some would advise suture plus reinforcement or 'augmentation' by the construction of an artificial ligament, but most surgeons prefer to await events and to reconstruct the ligament secondarily if significant disability persists after a prolonged period of rehabilitation. Concomitant lesions of the medial (or lateral) ligament or of a meniscus should, however, be dealt with surgically in the acute stage when appropriate.

Anterior cruciate tears of long standing are amenable to reconstructive surgery, but each case must be considered on its merits and a decision made to operate only if the disability clearly justifies it. It must be remembered, firstly, that some patients are able to lead an almost normal life, including moderate participation in sport, despite a persistently lax anterior cruciate ligament; and, secondly, that ligament reconstruction, though often affording improvement, seldom restores full stability. Moreover the result may deteriorate with time, because of stretching.

If reconstruction is decided upon, it may be by the substitution of a strip of aponeurosis or tendon (usually a strip from the patellar tendon). In many cases reconstruction of the medial (or lateral) ligament is required at the same time. Use has been made in the past of synthetic material as a substitute for the damaged ligament, but results have been less satisfactory than those from the use of homogenous material.

Posterior cruciate tears. Tears of the posterior cruciate ligament are amenable to reconstruction, which should, however, be undertaken only when the disability justifies it. If the posterior tibial spine has been avulsed with the ligament, the separated fragment may be fixed back in its bed with a screw.

After reconstruction of cruciate ligaments it is important that intensive exercises be practised in order to redevelop the quadriceps muscle. A powerful muscle can compensate to some extent for minor residual laxity of the joint.

Avulsion of the tibial spine

Rarely, a force acting through a cruciate ligament pulls a fragment of bone from the intercondylar ridge of the upper surface of the tibia, the ligament itself remaining intact. The bone fragment may be displaced slightly upwards, away from its bed. In most cases satisfactory reduction is achieved simply by extending the knee fully, and it is sufficient thereafter to immobilise the limb in a plaster for 4 weeks. If the bone fragment is more widely displaced and cannot be reduced by manipulation, it may have to be replaced at open operation and fixed in position by a small screw.

Strain of the medial or lateral ligament

A force that is insufficient to tear a ligament completely may cause a partial tear or strain. Either the medial or the lateral ligament (with the adjacent part of the capsule) may be affected. The medial ligament is strained by a force that abducts the tibia upon the femur, whereas the lateral ligament is strained by an adduction force. Strain of the medial ligament is much the more common— indeed, it is one of the most common of all knee injuries.

Clinical features

There is a history of an abduction or adduction injury. The knee is painful at the site of the injured ligament and may be noticed to be swollen. On examination there is localised tenderness on palpation over the affected ligament, either in its course or at its upper or lower attachment. Applying stress to the ligament may cause pain, but the knee is stable. There may be an effusion of fluid within the joint. The quadriceps muscle may be slightly wasted, but this is not a striking feature (compare torn meniscus). Flexion and extension of the knee are restricted by a few degrees because of pain when the ligament becomes taut.

Diagnosis

Strain of the medial ligament cannot always be differentiated with certainty from a tear of the medial meniscus at the first examination. Indeed, the two injuries may coexist. Arthroscopy may be needed, particularly to reveal the state of the meniscus. Without arthroscopy, the diagnosis will become clear clinically if the knee is observed at intervals over a few weeks. After a strain the fluid effusion (if any) is usually absorbed within 2 or 3 weeks, and full move-ment is regained in a similar time. If effusion and painful limitation of exten-sion persist for more than 3 weeks the diagnosis of strained ligament may have to be revised in favour of one of torn meniscus, and at that stage arthroscopy should be undertaken if it has not already been done.

Course

Strains of the medial (or lateral) ligament tend to heal slowly. It is common for pain to persist in decreasing degree for about 2 months, but eventual full recovery is to be expected.

Treatment

If pain and tenderness are severe a preliminary period of 2 weeks' rest in plaster (from groin to malleoli) should be advised. Thereafter, treatment should be by active exercises to redevelop the quadriceps muscle.

Pellegrini–Stieda's disease

In a few cases of incomplete avulsion of the medial ligament from the medial epicondyle of the femur, ossification occurs in the small haematoma that forms between the ligament and the femoral condyle. This condition is sometimes referred to as Pellegrini–Stieda's disease.

Clinically there is persistent discomfort at the medial side of the knee after an injury to the medial ligament. There are thickening and slight tenderness over the site of attachment of the ligament to the medial femoral epicondyle. Radiographs show a thin plaque of new bone close to the medial epicondyle.

Treatment is by active mobilising and muscle-strengthening exercises.

TEARS OF THE MENISCI OF THE KNEE

Injuries of the menisci (semilunar cartilages) are common in men under the age of 45 years. A tear is usually caused by a twisting force with the knee semi-flexed or flexed. It is usually a football or other sporting injury, but it is also common among men who work in a squatting position. The medial meniscus is torn much more often than the lateral.

Pathology

There are three types of tear (Fig. 15.17). All begin as a longitudinal split (Fig. 15.18A). If this extends throughout the length of the meniscus it becomes a

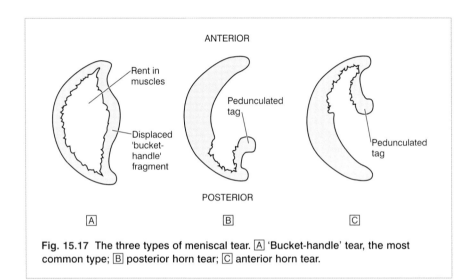

Fig. 15.17 The three types of meniscal tear. A 'Bucket-handle' tear, the most common type; B posterior horn tear; C anterior horn tear.

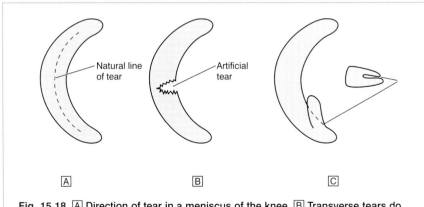

Fig. 15.18 A Direction of tear in a meniscus of the knee. B Transverse tears do not occur naturally; a tear such as this is always an artefact. C Horizontal tear of degenerative medial meniscus.

'bucket-handle' tear, in which the fragments remain attached at both ends (Fig. 15.17A). This is much the most common type. The 'bucket-handle' (that is, the central fragment) is displaced towards the middle of the joint, so that the condyle of the femur rolls upon the tibia through the rent in the meniscus. Since the femoral condyle is so shaped that it requires most space when the knee is straight, the chief effect of a displaced 'bucket-handle' is that it limits full extension. This block to full extension—a characteristic sign—is referred to loosely as 'locking'.

If the initial longitudinal tear emerges at the concave border of the meniscus a pedunculated tag is formed. In posterior horn tear the fragment remains attached at its posterior horn (Fig. 15.17B); in anterior horn tear it remains attached at its anterior horn (Fig. 15.17C). A transverse tear through the meniscus is usually an artefact, produced at the time of operation (Fig. 15.18B).

The menisci of the knee are almost avascular: so when they are torn there is not an effusion of blood into the joint, but there is an effusion of synovial fluid, secreted in response to the injury. Major tears of the menisci do not heal spontaneously.

Clinical features of a torn medial meniscus

The patient is aged 18–50 years. The history is characteristic, especially with 'bucket-handle' tears. In consequence of a twisting injury the patient falls and has pain at the antero-medial aspect of the joint. He is unable to continue what he was doing, or does so only with difficulty. He is unable to straighten the knee fully. The next day he notices that the whole knee is swollen. He rests the knee. After about 2 weeks the swelling lessens, the knee seems to go straight again, and he resumes his activities. Within weeks or months the knee suddenly gives way again during a twisting movement, with pain and subsequent swelling as before. Similar incidents occur repeatedly.

Locking. By 'locking' is meant inability to extend the knee fully. It is not a true jamming of the joint because there is a free range of flexion. Locking is a common and important feature of torn medial meniscus, but the limitation of extension is often so slight that it is not noticed by the patient and may, indeed, be overlooked by the surgeon. Persistent locking can occur only in 'bucket-handle' tears: tag tears cause momentary catching but not true locking in the accepted sense.

On examination in the recent stage of a meniscus injury the typical features are effusion of fluid, wasting of the quadriceps muscle, local tenderness at the level of the joint antero-medially, and (characteristically in 'bucket-handle' tears) limitation of the last few degrees of extension by a springy resistance, with sharp antero-medial pain if passive extension is forced.

In the 'silent' phase between attacks there are often no signs other than wasting of the quadriceps muscle.

Clinical features of a torn lateral meniscus

The features are broadly similar, but the clinical picture is often less clearly defined. The history may be vague, but a precipitating injury is always recalled. Pain is at the lateral rather than the medial side of the joint, but it is often poorly localised.

Plain radiographs are normal, whether the tear be of the medial or of the lateral meniscus.

Fig. 15.19 A Arthroscopic image showing tear of medial meniscus with displaced 'bucket handle' (arrow). B Magnetic resonance image (MRI) of knee joint showing a tear in the posterior horn of the medial meniscus.

Diagnosis

In the 'silent' phase clinical diagnosis often depends largely upon the history. Plain radiographs are normal, whether the tear be of the medial or of the lateral meniscus. The surgeon should be very cautious in diagnosing a torn meniscus unless there is a clear history of injury and unless there have been recurrent incidents, each followed by synovial effusion. Often a period of observation is required before the clinical diagnosis becomes reasonably certain. If a meniscal tear is suspected, arthroscopy may be expected to clinch the diagnosis (Fig. 15.19A). Magnetic resonance imaging is also diagnostic (Fig. 15.19B) in a high proportion of cases and, where available, is preferable as a non-invasive investigation.

Late effects

Long continued internal derangement from a torn meniscus predisposes to the later development of osteoarthritis. Arthritis may also develop years after a meniscus has been removed.

Treatment

Once the diagnosis is established the correct treatment is to excise the displaced fragment of the meniscus, or in some cases the whole meniscus. With the rapid advances that have taken place in arthroscopic surgery, most meniscus excisions are now carried out arthroscopically, without formal opening of the joint. Arthroscopic techniques have now been developed to allow repair of meniscal tears, though this is only appropriate for fresh injuries and in expert hands. The long-term results of this method remain uncertain.

Treatment of the locked knee. Manipulation under anaesthesia is the standard practice in the acute stage when there is a marked block to extension. But it cannot be expected that manipulation will restore the displaced 'bucket-handle' to its normal position: it merely extends the tear longitudinally and thereby allows the 'bucket-handle' fragment to move further towards the middle of the joint—that is, to the intercondylar region. In this position the displaced fragment allows greater freedom of joint movement, but completely full extension is seldom restored. Manipulation is therefore worthwhile only in so far as it increases the patient's comfort while awaiting admission for operation.

Horizontal tear of degenerate medial meniscus

The meniscal tears described above are uncommon in patients over the age of 50 years, when the menisci begin to show degenerative changes. But a degenerate meniscus is liable to suffer a different type of lesion. The medial meniscus in particular may split horizontally (Fig. 15.18C) at a point near its attachment to the medial ligament of the knee. Such a split is usually of small dimensions, and because there is no separation of the fragments natural healing can occur.

Clinically there is troublesome and persistent pain at the medial aspect of the knee at the joint level. The pain may be noticed after a minor injury, but often it seems to come on spontaneously, without any recognised incident. In the early stages there is usually a small effusion of fluid into the joint.

Treatment should be expectant at first, by bandaging and quadriceps exercises. In most cases the symptoms resolve in the course of several months. In the occasional case in which they fail to do so, arthroscopy with trimming or excision of the meniscus should be advised.

TRAUMATIC EFFUSIONS IN THE KNEE

The knee commonly becomes distended with fluid after an injury. The fluid may be a clear serous effusion, blood or, occasionally, pus. A purulent effusion is easily distinguished by pyrexia and general constitutional disturbance associated with local signs of inflammation. The problem that usually arises is to distinguish clinically between a clear serous effusion and a haemarthrosis.

A serous effusion occurs after an injury that damages some part of the synovial tissues but does not tear any vascular structure. It occurs regularly after tears of the menisci and often after strains or contusions of the capsule or ligaments. The characteristics of a clear serous effusion are that it forms slowly over a period of 24 hours or so and seldom becomes very tense.

A haemarthrosis, on the other hand, is caused by an injury that tears the vascular tissues of the joint, and it is observed therefore after complete ruptures of the ligaments or capsule, after fractures of the patella or of the articular surfaces of the femur or tibia, and after avulsion of the quadriceps tendon from the patella. The features of a haemarthrosis are that it forms rapidly, reaching a maximum within a few hours of the injury, and that the effusion is tense. The overlying skin is warmer than normal. Because of the greater tension, a haemarthrosis causes more severe pain than a clear serous effusion.

Treatment

Clear serous effusions should usually be allowed to absorb spontaneously. Blood effusions that are tense and causing severe pain should be reduced by aspiration, and controlled thereafter by firm bandaging and immobilisation. Later arthroscopy may be required to identify, and if necessary treat, the source of the haemarthrosis.

16 | Leg and ankle

CLASSIFICATION

Fractures of the tibia and fibula

[1]	Fractures of the condyles of the tibia
[2]	Fractures of the shafts of the tibia and fibula
[2]	Fracture of the shaft of the tibia alone
[2]	Fracture of the fibula alone
[3]	Fractures and fracture-dislocations about the ankle

Soft-tissue injuries about the ankle

Rupture of the lateral ligaments of the ankle
Strain of the lateral ligaments
Rupture of the calcaneal tendon

The most common injuries to be encountered in this region are undoubtedly those about the ankle—often fractures of the lateral or medial malleolus or of both malleoli, or strain of the ligaments of the ankle—particularly the lateral ligament. Also prevalent in this region are fractures of the shafts of the tibia and fibula, very often caused by motor-cycling accidents and sporting injuries.

FRACTURES OF THE TIBIA AND FIBULA

FRACTURES OF THE CONDYLES OF THE TIBIA

Most fractures of the tibial condyles involve only the lateral condyle. Less often the medial condyle is fractured alone, and occasionally both condyles are fractured together.

FRACTURE OF THE LATERAL TIBIAL CONDYLE

The common fracture of the lateral condyle is caused by a force that abducts the tibia upon the femur while the foot is fixed on the ground[1] (Fig. 16.1). An example of this mechanism is seen when the bumper of a car strikes the outer side of the knee of a pedestrian. So often is this type of accident responsible that

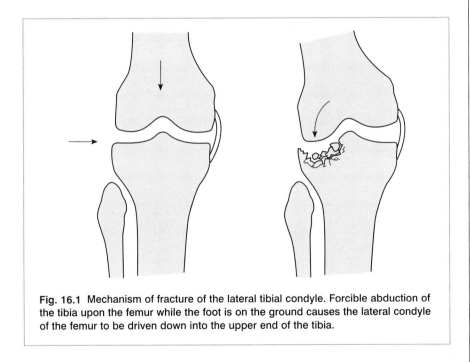

Fig. 16.1 Mechanism of fracture of the lateral tibial condyle. Forcible abduction of the tibia upon the femur while the foot is on the ground causes the lateral condyle of the femur to be driven down into the upper end of the tibia.

[1] A force that abducts the tibia upon the femur is also the cause of injuries of the medial ligament of the knee (p. 258), In general, an abduction force will cause a condylar fracture rather than a ligamentous injury if the foot is bearing weight upon the ground at the time of the injury-especially in an elderly person with soft bones. A similar force applied when the foot is off the ground is more likely to injure the medial ligament. Occasionally the two injuries are associated.

Leg and ankle

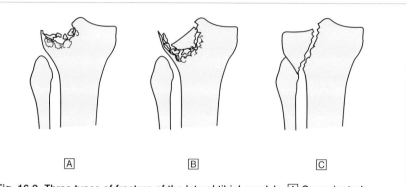

Fig. 16.2 Three types of fracture of the lateral tibial condyle. [A] Comminuted compression fracture. [B] Depressed plateau fracture without severe fragmentation. [C] Oblique shearing fracture.

Fig. 16.3 A typical depressed fracture of the lateral tibial condyle with fragmentation of the articular surface.

the injury has been called a bumper fracture. Many such patients are women past middle age, which suggests that osteoporosis may be an additional factor predisposing to fracture.

The pattern of the fracture may be of three types:

1. *Comminuted compression fracture.* This is the most common pattern. The lateral tibial condyle, including its articular surface, is crushed and fragmented by the impact of the lateral condyle of the femur which is driven down into it (Figs 16.1, 16.2A & 16.3).
2. *Depressed plateau type.* This is less common than the comminuted compression fracture. A large part of the articular surface of the lateral condyle is depressed into the shell of the bone but remains largely intact as a single piece, without marked fragmentation (Fig. 16.2B).
3. *Oblique shearing fracture.* This is the least common type. The whole or a large part of the condyle is sheared off in one piece through an oblique fracture (Fig. 16.2C).

Fig. 16.4 Ⓐ Radiograph and Ⓑ CT scan of depressed fracture of the lateral tibial condyle.

Treatment

The treatment depends largely upon the type of fracture as seen radiographically. Plain radiographs may fail to reveal the full extent of the damage to the articular surface and CT scans (Fig. 16.4B) are increasingly employed to allow appropriate treatment planning, particularly when surgical intervention is contemplated.

Comminuted compression fracture. This forms the largest group (Fig. 16.3). Because the articular surface of the condyle is broken into innumerable tiny pieces, many of which are crushed down into the underlying soft cancellous bone, it is hardly practicable to restore the articular surface to its original smooth state. On the other hand further displacement is unlikely to occur because the forces acting through the knee under conditions of treatment will be small compared with the force that caused the injury. The fracture, which is through spongy bone, will always unite readily. Thus the method of treatment now widely practised is to accept the displacement, to avoid rigid immobilisation and to encourage active movements of the knee from the beginning. It may, indeed, be hoped that movement of the joint, at a stage when the granulation tissue covering the broken surfaces is still pliable, will help to restore a smooth articular surface.

Initially, the patient is confined to bed, and if a tense haemarthrosis has formed the blood-stained fluid is aspirated. A removable plaster shell is constructed to protect the knee from unguarded and possibly painful lateral movements at night. During the day the plaster splint is removed to allow active exercises. These are carried out under the supervision of a physiotherapist; they include exercises to restore the tone of the quadriceps and hamstring muscles, and flexion and extension movements of the knee. After recumbency for 2–4 weeks (according to the severity of the fracture) it is safe to allow walking with sticks without any external splintage. Thereafter rehabilitation may be continued on a regular basis in the gymnasium, usually with good results.

Cast-bracing. To avoid the risks of prolonged bed rest, many of these fractures are now treated by cast-bracing (functional bracing) (see p. 40). The brace protects the knee sufficiently to allow weight-bearing within 1 or 2 weeks, and at the same time knee movements are permitted by the hinge.

Depressed plateau fracture without fragmentation. In this group an attempt should usually be made to restore the articular surface of the tibial condyle to something approaching normal. A 'window' is cut in the antero-lateral cortex of the tibia a little below the level of the joint. Through this aperture the depressed fragment is pushed up from below by a broad punch, until the articular fragment is flush with the surrounding cartilage, as confirmed by inspection through an upward prolongation of the incision that opens the knee joint or through an arthroscope. The cavity in the lower part of the tibial condyle is then packed firmly with cancellous bone chips to hold the fragment in position. To prevent redisplacement of the reconstructed surface, the tibial condyle may be further buttressed by a broad plate fixed with transverse screws (Fig. 16.5).

Oblique shearing fracture (Fig. 16.2C). This type of fracture lends itself well to operative reduction and internal fixation by a long cancellous screw. It is essential that the displaced fragment be replaced perfectly in its bed, to avoid any 'step' in the articular surface.

Comment. It is unfortunate that the fractures for which operation tends to be least rewarding—namely the comminuted compression type—are the most common. On the other hand, the victims of this type of fracture are often elderly, and the results of conservative treatment are usually adequate for their needs. Operation should generally be advised in those cases in which there is

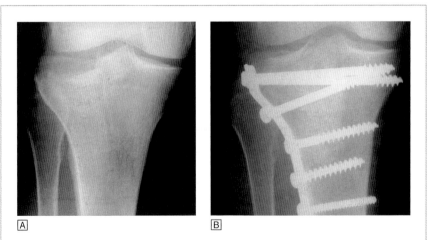

Fig. 16.5 Depressed plateau fracture of the lateral tibial condyle before A and after B elevation and buttressing with a plate and screws.

a chance of elevating a more-or-less intact articular surface to its normal position, except perhaps in patients of advanced age.

Complications
These are: (1) genu valgum, (2) joint stiffness and (3) late osteoarthritis.

Genu valgum. When there is some residual and irremediable depression of the lateral tibial condyle a minor degree of genu valgum is often unavoidable. In most cases it is insufficient to cause serious inconvenience and may therefore be accepted.

Stiffness of the knee. With treatment by early exercises it is surprising how quickly a good range of knee movement is regained; indeed, in the average case knee stiffness is not a serious problem. There are exceptions, however, and sometimes months of physiotherapy by active exercises are required before reasonable movement is restored. Manipulation under anaesthesia may sometimes be helpful.

Osteoarthritis. Because the damaged articular surface of the tibial condyle often remains irregular there is theoretically a risk of later osteoarthritis. However, when the articular damage is relatively slight, arthritis may take many years to reach the stage of causing severe disability, and because many patients with this injury are beyond middle age the need for active treatment of the arthritis may never arise.

In cases of severe painful post-traumatic osteoarthritis, operation may sometimes be justified: corrective osteotomy, by removal of a medial wedge from the upper end of the tibia, often gives adequate relief. Only occasionally is a more radical operation required: this may take the form of replacement arthroplasty or, exceptionally, arthrodesis.

Fracture of the medial tibial condyle

This injury, which is relatively uncommon, is virtually the mirror-image of fracture of the lateral condyle. Its features and treatment are comparable to those of lateral condylar fractures, and no special description is required.

FRACTURES OF THE SHAFTS OF THE TIBIA AND FIBULA

Most fractures in this region involve both the tibia and the fibula (Fig 16.6A), and the following description applies to such combined injuries. Fractures of the tibia alone and of the fibula alone will be considered in later sections.

Mechanism and displacement
Fractures of the shafts of the tibia and fibula may occur either from an angulatory force or from a rotational force. Fractures from an angulatory force tend to be transverse or of the short oblique type, and the fractures of tibia and fibula are at about the same level. Fractures from a rotational force are spiral, and at a widely different level in the two bones. Often the tibial fracture is at the junction of the middle and lowest thirds whereas the fibular fracture is near the junction of the middle and uppermost thirds. As a rule there is considerable displacement of the fragments, though undisplaced crack fractures are seen commonly in children.

Fig. 16.6 Typical fractures of the shafts of the tibia and fibula shown in antero-posterior and lateral radiographs before Ⓐ and after Ⓑ manipulative reduction and immobilisation in plaster.

Because the tibia is so close to the surface and so poorly protected by muscle, many fractures of its shaft are of the open (compound) type; indeed, the tibial shaft is more often the site of an open fracture than is any other bone.

In Britain motor-cycle accidents are by far the most common single cause of major fractures of the shafts of the tibia and fibula.

Treatment

In fresh fractures of both bones of the leg, attention should be concentrated solely on the fracture of the tibia. The fibular fracture may be disregarded because it always unites readily, and in any case the bone is of such secondary importance that the position of the fragments is immaterial. In contrast, the tibial fracture requires close supervision to ensure normal length and correct alignment. Imperfect end-to-end apposition of the fragments may be accepted provided the displacement is not enough to cause ugly deformity.

As with fractures of the shaft of the femur, conservative treatment should still be the method of choice whenever it is practicable. Indeed, there is less justification for abandoning conservative treatment in favour of operative fixation for these fractures than there is in the case of the femur, because during conservative treatment the patient is usually able to get about well in plaster, need not remain in hospital for long, and may often return to work while the leg is still in plaster or in a functional brace. Nevertheless, there should be no hesitation in advising operative fixation when the indications for it arise, and with the wider adoption of 'closed' intramedullary nailing the scope for operation is perhaps wider than it was a few years ago.

Fig. 16.7 Plaster used for fractures of the shafts of the tibia and fibula.

Standard method of conservative treatment. The accepted method of treatment is to reduce the fracture (when necessary) by closed manipulation (Fig. 16.6B) and to immobilise the limb in a full-length plaster. The knee is held slightly flexed to help to prevent rotation of the limb within the plaster and to facilitate walking and sitting. The ankle is held at a right angle, and the toes are left free (Fig. 16.7). The plaster may later be 'wedged' if necessary to correct an imperfection of alignment, by dividing it round two-thirds of its circumference at the level of the fracture and angulating it in the required direction before repairing the plaster. The plaster may need to be changed after 1 or 2 weeks as the initial soft-tissue swelling subsides, or if it becomes loose or uncomfortable.

If the fracture seems stable against redisplacement (as, for example, a transverse fracture) walking should be encouraged after 2 or 3 weeks, when the acute local reaction to the injury has settled down. For this purpose a walking heel or rocker (made from plaster, wood or rubber) may be applied to the sole of the plaster, or alternatively a canvas overboot may be provided. But if the pattern of fracture suggests that it is liable to redisplacement (for example, an oblique or spiral fracture), full unprotected weight-bearing on the affected leg should be deferred for about 6 weeks, though walking with crutches may be allowed earlier.

The plaster is retained until the tibial fracture is firmly united as shown by clinical and radiographic examination (Figs 2.4 & 2.5, p. 27), usually a matter of between 3 and 4 months. Thereafter active exercises are carried out under the supervision of a physiotherapist to restore a full range of knee, ankle and foot movements and to redevelop the muscles.

Cast-bracing. In many cases the period of full immobilisation of the knee and ankle may be reduced by substituting a carefully applied functional brace (see

Fig. 16.8 Functional brace (cast brace) with ankle hinges used for selected healing fractures of the tibia.

p. 40) for the full plaster-often about 4–6 weeks from the time of injury. A full-length brace (see Fig. 15.5) incorporates hinges at the knee, and optionally also at the ankle. Later, in the case of a lower tibial fracture the brace may leave the knee free (Fig. 16.8). The use of cast-bracing has been extended with the advent of new casting materials. Cast-bracing may possibly have additional advantages in stimulating union by restoring physiological forces through the bone.

Caution. As with all functional bracing, careful supervision is required to ensure that angulation does not occur, from premature or unskilful application of the brace.

Operative treatment: internal fixation. Internal (operative) fixation is required mainly when the fracture cannot be reduced adequately by manipulation, or when plaster alone fails to maintain an acceptable position of the fragments. Operation is required much more often for oblique or spiral fractures, which always tend to be unstable, than for transverse fractures (Fig. 1.3, p. 6).

The method of internal fixation must be chosen to suit each individual fracture: there is no universal method. The introduction of the sophisticated instrumentation and technology of the AO system led to widespread use of plates and screws to provide more rigid compression fixation for tibial shaft fractures. Initially this method was preferred to intramedullary nailing because of the better control of rotational stability. Since the advent of the newer `locking nails', allowing the insertion of proximal and distal cross-screws (Fig. 16.10) to control rotation, the use of intramedullary fixation has increased. It is now the method of choice for the fixation of most tibial shaft fractures, since it requires less soft tissue deception at the fracture site, reducing the risk of infection or non-union.

Plate and screws. Plating has long been an accepted and widely used method of fixation of a fracture of the tibial shaft (Fig. 16.9). The plate is nearly always of metal, usually an inert surgical grade of stainless steel. After fixation by a

Fig. 16.9 Tibial fracture before $\boxed{A}$ and after $\boxed{B}$ being fixed internally by metal plate and screws.

plate, the additional support of a plaster may be advisable until union is shown radiologically. The use of compression plates was discussed on page 43.

Intramedullary nail. Intramedullary nailing is now used increasingly in preference to plating, especially for fractures near the middle of the tibial shaft without much comminution (Fig. 16.10). It may present difficulties when the fracture is severely comminuted, though the newer types of nail, which have perforations to allow cross-screwing proximally or distally, have gone some way to overcoming them. Nailing is generally unsuitable for the management of fractures close to the upper or lower articular surface. Intramedullary nailing offers the advantage of stronger fixation than that provided by other methods of internal fixation, including plating; so the additional support of a plaster is seldom required and early weight-bearing may be encouraged. Furthermore, in cases suitable for 'closed' nailing (see below) the risk of infection is reduced to a minimum. The nail may be left free in the bone, or it may be locked at the ends by cross-screws ('locking screws') driven through perforations in the nail.

Whenever possible, the operation should be done by the closed technique, without exposing the fracture. Reduction may have to be aided by mechanical traction through a Steinmann pin in the lower end of the tibia. With the knee flexed, a long guide wire is introduced into the tibia from above through a short incision medial to the patellar tendon and advanced as far as the fracture. When reduction has been secured and checked radiographically the guide wire is driven across the fracture into the distal fragment. The medullary canal is reamed over the guide wire to the appropriate diameter, usually about 12 mm, and a nail of corresponding size is driven home. If a locking nail is used, one

Fig. 16.10 Transverse fractures of the shafts of the tibia and fibula before A and B after being treated by intramedullary nailing of the tibia.

or two cross-screws are inserted through the bone to engage the corresponding holes in the nail.

If closed reduction and nailing are not practicable it is necessary to use the open method. The fracture is exposed and the fragments are realigned under direct vision.

Function of the knee is not disturbed by entering the nail through the inter-condylar ridge because this region of the tibia does not form part of the articular surface.

Treatment by external fixation. The technique of external fixation in general was described on page 41. The method is particularly suitable for open fractures in which the risk of infection may preclude internal fixation, and for fractures that are already infected. At least two pins, and preferably three, are inserted in each main fragment. They are left protruding and fixed to a rigid bar on the antero-medial (subcutaneous) aspect of the leg (Fig. 16.11). More rigid fixation can be gained by using longer transfixion pins passed through the bone and incorporated on both sides in an external frame, but this makes early mobilisation of the patient more difficult.

Treatment by continuous traction. If the patient is confined to bed on account of other injuries there is an occasional place for treatment by sustained traction with the limb resting upon a Braun's frame. Traction is applied through a transfixion pin in the lower end of the tibia. The use of a calcaneal pin for leg traction is to be discouraged because the pin-track is more liable to troublesome infection or residual tenderness.

Fig. 16.11 [A] Radiograph of tibial fracture with 'Orthofix' external applicator applied. [B] 'Orthofix' fixator used in the treatment of an open tibial fracture.

Complications

Infection. Because of the frequency with which tibial fractures are associated with a communicating skin wound, contamination and consequent osteomyelitis are more common than in any other bone. Nevertheless, cases of serious infection are seen much less often now than they were some years ago, because contamination is reduced by prompt cleansing of the wound and excision of devitalised tissue (p. 48), and because antibiotics are used prophylactically in the early days after the injury.

Established infection is indicated by persistent pyrexia and a 'suppurative' odour over the wound. In that event the plaster must be split and free drainage provided—if it is not already established—by opening up the wound. Later, fragments of dead bone (sequestra) may have to be removed. When the infection has been overcome, healing may be hastened by applying split-skin grafts to the granulating surface. In cases of serious infection, union of the fracture is generally delayed or prevented (Fig. 4.1, p. 53).

Delayed union and non-union. Whereas most tibial fractures unite readily, a small proportion may be very obstinate and may still be freely mobile 3 or 4 months after the injury. In that event surgical intervention is usually to be advised, provided the skin is healthy. In most cases a bone-grafting operation is recommended.

In the technique that is commonly used when the fragments are already in acceptable apposition and alignment, slivers of cancellous bone are inserted beneath the periosteum and the fracture itself is not disturbed. If it is necessary to adjust the position of the fragments, cancellous grafting may be combined with the use of an intramedullary nail to provide rigidity.

There is no need to graft the fibula, which always unites readily: indeed, it is sometimes necessary to divide the fibula before the tibial fragments can be brought into exact apposition. In practice an intact fibula may hinder union of the tibia, because if there has been slight absorption of the tibial fractures the fibula acts as a strut, holding the tibial fragments apart.

If persistent infection makes metallic internal fixation and bone grafting inadvisable, external fixation may be used as an alternative. This provides stability against refracture while allowing access to the infected bone and soft tissues for continued surgical or conservative treatment. Bone grafting should not be attempted while infection is still present in the bone at the site of non-union.

If non-union defies all these methods, a course of treatment by electrical stimulation (p. 56) may be considered.

Mal-union. With the general improvement in the standard of fracture treatment, mal-union has become uncommon. Nevertheless, cases are still seen in which union of a tibial fracture has occurred with overlap and consequent shortening, or with angulation (sometimes resulting from premature or injudicious use of a cast-brace). In most cases it is wise to accept the disability if the deformity is slight, but if an angular deformity is severe it may be advisable to correct it by osteotomy of the tibia and fibula, especially since severe mal-alignment predisposes to the later development of osteoarthritis of the knee or ankle.

Impairment of the vascular supply. A displaced tibial fracture—particularly one involving the proximal half of the bone–may damage a major branch of the popliteal artery, with consequent obstruction of the arterial flow and risk of serious ischaemia below the lesion. This disaster demands emergency operation to repair the injured vessel (see p. 62). Another important cause of vascular impairment is a build-up of pressure within a fascial compartment (anterior, lateral or posterior) from oedema occurring in the closed space, a condition that should be suspected if complaint of severe pain is associated with notable impairment of toe movement (Compartment syndrome, see p. 63). In this event immediate operative decompression of the compartment is imperative. Constriction from overtight dressings or plaster may precipitate a similar emergency.

In this connection it must be stressed once again that it is essential to examine for signs of circulatory impairment or peripheral nerve injury when the patient is first received for treatment. The condition of the circulation in the toes must be watched closely during the first 2 days after an injury to, or operation on, the leg.

Injury to a major nerve. A displaced fracture of the tibia or fibula may damage a major nerve trunk—notably the common peroneal nerve or the tibial nerve just below the knee, and the tibial nerve in fractures of the lower quarter of the tibia. The general management of nerve injuries complicating fractures was discussed on page 64.

FRACTURE OF THE SHAFT OF THE TIBIA ALONE

Fracture of the tibial shaft without a fracture of the fibula is relatively uncommon. Displacement tends to be less severe than in fractures of both bones.

Treatment
The principles of treatment are the same as for fractures of the tibia and fibula together. In most cases the fragments can be held adequately by a full-length plaster (Fig. 16.7). Sometimes the intact fibula acts to the disadvantage of the tibial fracture, because it may prevent the fracture surfaces from coming together in close apposition, or hinder the restoration of normal alignment. If this strut-like effect of the intact fibula seems to be provoking deformity or delaying union a short length of the fibula should be excised (see p. 280).

Fatigue fracture of the tibia

Rarely, a crack fracture may occur through the shaft of the tibia from repeated minor stresses rather than from a major injury. This type of fracture—more common in the metatarsal bones—is termed a fatigue or stress fracture (see p. 14).

There is usually a history of unaccustomed repetitive activity, such as prolonged walking, running or dancing, preceding the onset of symptoms. It is a well recognised complication of excessive marching in new military recruits. The patient complains of pain over the tibia, and walking becomes difficult or impossible. There is local tenderness over the site of fracture, and radiographs show a faint transverse crack (Fig. 1.10, p. 15). Union occurs readily. Protection for a few weeks in a full-length walking plaster is advised.

FRACTURE OF THE FIBULA ALONE

The shaft of the fibula is seldom broken without the tibia, or without a simultaneous ankle injury in the form of tibio-fibular diastasis (p. 289). Thus the ankle should always be radiographed, whatever the level of the fibular fracture. When an isolated fracture of the fibular shaft does occur it is usually caused by a direct blow over the bone. Displacement is seldom severe. There is marked local tenderness over the site of the fracture, but since the tibia is intact the patient is able to continue walking, and on this account the fracture may be overlooked.

No special treatment is required except to relieve pain. For this purpose protection in a below-knee walking plaster for 3 weeks is usually sufficient.

Fatigue fracture of the fibula

Fatigue or stress fractures, though much more common in the metatarsals, are well recognised in the fibula. They usually affect the lowest third of the bone, but they may also occur at the middle or uppermost third. There is no history of sudden injury, and the patient seeks advice on account of spontaneous pain at the outer side of the leg, usually after an unusual amount of walking, running or dancing. Radiographs at first may show no more than a faint hairline crack across the bone, but later the site of fracture is made evident by surrounding callus.

FRACTURES AND FRACTURE–DISLOCATIONS ABOUT THE ANKLE

The bones forming the ankle mortise are injured more often than any other bone except the lower end of the radius. Many distinct varieties of these fractures and fracture–dislocations are recognised. In the past they were often grouped together loosely under the general title 'Pott's[2] fracture' and this term is still used occasionally.

Mechanism of injury and patterns of fracture

Most fractures about the ankle involve either the lateral malleolus or the medial malleolus, or both malleoli together, with or without subluxation or dislocation of the talus from its normal position within the tibio-fibular mortise. The most severe injuries are those in which the inferior articular surface of the tibia is shattered.

Fractures and dislocations of the ankle usually result from one of three injury mechanisms; an abduction or lateral rotation force or a combination of both; an adduction force; or a vertical compression force. The patterns of fracture caused by each of these three types of violence are illustrated diagrammatically in Fig. 16.12.

In practice it will be found that there are seven distinct patterns of fracture or fracture–dislocations to be considered from the point of view of treatment, and these will be discussed individually in the following pages:

1. Isolated fracture of the lateral malleolus
2. Isolated fracture of the medial malleolus
3. Fracture of the lateral malleolus with lateral shift of the talus
4. Fractures of both malleoli with displacement of the talus
5. Tibio-fibular diastasis
6. Posterior marginal fracture of the tibia with posterior displacement of the talus
7. Vertical compression fracture of the lower articular surface of the tibia.

General principles of treatment

In fractures without displacement it is usually sufficient to protect the ankle in a below-knee walking plaster (Fig. 16.13) for 3–6 weeks, depending upon the nature of the injury. In such cases the purpose of providing protection by a plaster splint is predominantly for the relief of pain.

In fractures with displacement the necessary action must be taken to ensure: (1) that the tibia and fibula are in normal relationship to one another at their lower ends, to form the ankle mortise and (2) that the talus is restored to its normal relationship with the tibio-fibular mortise. Reduction is effected by

---

[2] Percival Pott (1714-1788), a surgeon of St Bartholomew's Hospital, London, described in 1769 a fracture of the ankle region. The precise anatomical nature of the injury he described is uncertain, though it is clear from his description that he was referring to a fracture of the lower end of the fibula with lateral displacement of the talus. Pott himself suffered an open fracture of the lower leg, but this was almost certainly a fracture of the shaft of the tibia and had nothing to do with the ankle injury that bears his name.

manipulation under anaesthesia, the talus and the displaced malleolar fragment or fragments being restored to position by firm pressure in a direction opposite to the direction of displacement. Thereafter the reduction must be maintained until union is well advanced, usually a matter of 8–10 weeks. In many cases sufficient immobilisation is afforded by a closely fitting plaster; but because in these unstable fractures there is always a risk of redisplacement within the plaster, check radiographs should be obtained a week after the initial reduction to show whether or not a satisfactory position has been maintained.

When adequate reduction, with normal relationships between tibia and fibula and talus, cannot be maintained by plaster alone, operative fixation is required. The usual technique is to secure the fragments in perfect position by screws or a plate. In the first 2 weeks after operation many surgeons allow the ankle to remain free to allow mobilising exercises; at the same time elevation is encouraged to reduce swelling. Thereafter it may be advisable to protect the ankle in a below-knee plaster (Fig. 16.13) for 6–8 weeks, and this may permit walking at an early stage.

Complications

The simpler types of ankle injury are almost free from complications, and perfect function should always be restored. The more serious fracture-dislocations may be complicated by: (1) stiffness of the ankle, (2) persistent swelling from oedema of the soft tissues, and (3) later osteoarthritis. All these complications are most likely to occur when the articular surface of the ankle mortise has been damaged by the fracture, or when there is persistent displacement of the talus.

Persistent swelling and stiffness of the ankle. When the plaster is first removed there is a tendency to gravitational oedema, which may hinder the restoration of a full range of movement. Oedema may be controlled to some extent by crepe bandages or an elastic sock, but reliance should be placed mainly on exercises to restore muscle tone, with elevation of the limb when the patient is at rest. Oedema and stiffness are usually more troublesome in elderly patients than in the young.

A more serious problem from swelling and stiffness arises in reflex sympathetic dystrophy or Sudeck's post-traumatic osteodystrophy. In this condition, which is possibly related to sympathetic overaction, severe oedema with glazing of the overlying skin is associated with pain and obstinate stiffness not only of the ankle joint itself but also of the joints of the foot. Treatment by elevation, and intensive exercises under the supervision of a physiotherapist, must be prolonged. In an intractable case sympathetic blockade by intravenous infusions of guanethidine may be required (see p. 68).

Osteoarthritis. If a fracture involving the articular surface of the ankle mortise is not reduced perfectly so that the joint surfaces are smooth and congruous, wear-and-tear will be accelerated and osteoarthritis will develop months or years later (Fig. 4.13, p. 71). The greater the irregularity of the tibial articular surface, the more rapidly will degenerative changes occur.

Once established, osteoarthritis of the ankle does not respond well to conservative treatment, and if the disability is severe the most satisfactory treatment is to eliminate the joint by arthrodesis. Replacement arthroplasty, by the insertion of tibial and talar components, has been undertaken but the long-term results have been disappointing; in view of the generally excellent results obtained from arthrodesis, arthroplasty cannot yet be recommended.

Mechanism	Moderate violence

A Lateral rotation and/or abduction

① Shearing fracture of lateral malleolus

② Avulsion fracture of medial malleolus

B Adduction

⑦ Strain of lateral ligament

⑧ Shearing fracture of medial malleolus

⑨ Avulsion fracture of lateral malleolus

C Vertical compression

⑬ Anterior marginal fracture of tibia+anterior shift of talus

Fig. 16.12 In general, ankle fractures occur from three types of violence: A an abduction or lateral rotation force or a combination of both (the most common type); B an adduction force; or C a vertical compression force. The patterns of fracture caused by each of these three types of violence are shown here diagrammatically.

Severe violence			Additional displacement if momentum drives tibia forwards
③ Fracture lateral malleolus rupture medial ligament+lateral shift of talus	④ Fracture lateral and medial malleoli+ lateral shift of talus	⑤ Tibio-fibular diastasis. Rupture of tibio-fibular and medial ligaments +fracture shaft of fibula +lateral shift of talus	⑥ Posterior marginal fracture of tibial articular surface +posterior shift of talus
⑩ Complete rupture of lateral ligament	⑪ Fracture medial and lateral malleoli + medial shift of talus		⑫ Posterior marginal fracture of tibial articular surface +posterior shift of talus
⑭ Comminuted fracture of tibial articular surface+fracture of fibula+upward displacement of talus			

Fig. 16.12 (Cont'd).

Fig. 16.13 Below-knee plaster as used for most ankle fractures and for certain fractures of the foot. The ankle is held at about a right angle, and the position of the foot is neutral between inversion and eversion. The toes are left free to allow active movement. In the example shown a plaster rocker has been applied beneath the sole to facilitate walking: a rubber heel may be used for the same purpose.

Isolated fracture of the lateral malleolus

(Diagrams 1 and 9 in Fig. 16.12)
The lateral malleolus may be sheared off by an abduction or lateral rotation force (the usual cause), or avulsed by an adduction force. In the group under consideration there is no displacement of the talus because the medial malleolus and the medial ligament are intact. Nor is there usually any significant displacement of the malleolar fragment (Fig. 16.14).

Treatment
Treatment is required mainly to relieve pain and to restore function. Immobilisation is not essential to union, but a period of 3 weeks or so in a walking plaster is nevertheless usually desirable to relieve pain. Thereafter treatment is by active exercises to restore ankle and foot movements and muscle tone.

Isolated fracture of the medial malleolus

(Diagrams 2 and 8 in Fig. 16.12)
This may be regarded as the 'mirror-image' of the injury just described. It is much less common. The malleolus may be sheared off by an adduction force or

Fig. 16.14 Undisplaced fracture of the lateral malleolus. The oblique line of the fracture is seen through the shadow of the tibia in the lateral projection. (This injury corresponds to diagram 1 in Fig. 16.12.)

avulsed by an abduction force. The fracture is sometimes no more than a crack, but very often the malleolar fragment is displaced, with consequent loss of the smooth articular contour of the ankle mortise.

A notable feature of displaced fractures of the medial malleolus is that a fringe of periosteum may be turned in between the separated bone fragment and the main body of the bone, preventing accurate reduction by manipulation, and hindering union.

Treatment

The principle of treatment should be to rely upon conservative treatment by immobilisation in plaster if the malleolar fragment is not displaced or if perfect reduction can be secured by manipulation, but to resort to operation if perfect reduction cannot be secured by manipulation. It is important that the fragment be replaced perfectly, to ensure a smooth articular contour. In practice most of these fractures—other than simple cracks—do require operative reduction and internal fixation, which is easily effected by a long transfixion screw driven upwards from the tip of the malleolus. After the operation—or sometimes after a 2 weeks' period of rest during which mobilising exercises are encouraged—the ankle is immobilised in a below-knee plaster until union is well advanced (usually about 8 weeks). Walking in the plaster is allowed at an early stage.

Fracture of the lateral malleolus with lateral displacement of the talus

(Diagram 3 in Fig. 16.12)
The cause is an abduction or lateral rotation force. The medial malleolus is intact but the medial (deltoid) ligament is torn; otherwise lateral displacement of the talus could not occur. The shift of the talus is judged best from the width

Leg and ankle

Fig. 16.15 A Fracture of the lateral malleolus and lateral shift of the talus with the malleolar fragment. The widening of the joint space at the medial side, between the talus and the medial malleolus, indicates that the medial ligament is torn and the talus shifted. The displacement is slight but it must nevertheless be corrected. B Radiograph after reduction and immobilisation in plaster. (This injury corresponds to diagram 3 in Fig. 16.12.)

of the joint space between talus and medial malleolus. Normally this is equal to the space in the weight-bearing part of the joint; so if it is widened it follows that the talus must be displaced (Fig. 16.15A).

Treatment

Accurate reduction is essential to ensure congruous joint surfaces, and it can be achieved easily by strong inward pressure upon the lateral malleolus. In most cases the reduction can be held satisfactorily by a closely fitting plaster, in which walking may be permitted after the first few days (Figs 16.13 & 16.15B). The plaster should be retained for about 8 weeks, after which rehabilitation is continued by active exercises.

After this injury it is essential that check radiographs be obtained a week after reduction of the fracture. If check radiographs show that redisplacement has occurred despite close moulding of the plaster about the malleoli, operation should be advised. The lateral malleolus may be secured in position by a long screw driven obliquely medially and upwards from its lateral surface into the tibia, or by fixation of the fibular fragments with a small contoured plate held by screws. Post-operative management is the same as for fractures of the medial malleolus.

Fracture of both malleoli with lateral displacement of the talus

(Diagrams 4 and 11 in Fig. 16.12)
This injury is usually caused by an abduction or lateral rotation force, and is then merely a variation of the injury just described (Fig. 16.12, diagram 4), the

Fig. 16.16 Fracture of the medial and lateral malleoli with lateral displacement of the talus. A Before reduction. B After reduction and internal fixation of the medial malleolus with a screw and of the fibular fracture with a plate and screws, with one long screw holding the fibula to the tibia.

medial malleolus being avulsed instead of the ligament torn. In that case the malleolar fragments and the talus are displaced laterally (Fig. 16.16A). The same type of injury, but with medial displacement, occurs less commonly from an adduction force (Fig. 16.12, diagram 11).

Treatment

These fractures are difficult to reduce accurately by manipulation, and even when well reduced they are difficult to hold in position by plaster alone. Operation is therefore usually advised. In most cases it is sufficient to fix the medial malleolus back into position by a long transfixion screw (Fig. 16.16B): this automatically holds the talus and the lateral malleolus in correct relationship because both the medial and the lateral ligaments are intact. (In effect, fixation of the medial malleolus converts the fracture to that shown in diagram 1 in Figure 16.12.) But there can be no objection to fixation of the lateral malleolus also by screws or a plate, and some surgeons prefer to do this to ensure greater stability (Fig. 16.16).

Post-operative management is the same as for fractures of the medial malleolus alone.

Diastasis of the inferior tibio-fibular joint

(Diagram 5 in Fig. 16.12)

If violence acting laterally in an abduction injury is withstood by the lateral malleolus the brunt of the force falls upon the inferior tibio-fibular ligament and may rupture it, with consequent tibio-fibular diastasis (Fig. 16.12, diagram 5). The talus is displaced laterally with the lower end of the fibula, the medial ligament being ruptured or the medial malleolus avulsed, and the fibula is

Fig. 16.17 Tibio-fibular diastasis. The inferior tibio-fibular ligament and the medial ligament of the ankle have been torn, allowing lateral displacement of the fibula and the talus Ⓐ. This injury is always accompanied by a high fracture of the shaft of the fibula, which in this case was at its upper end Ⓑ. Ⓒ Shows the condition after reduction and fixation by a long screw. (This injury corresponds to diagram 5 in Fig. 16.12.)

fractured above the level of the inferior tibio-fibular ligament, often high up in the shaft (Fig. 16.17B).

Diagnosis

Slight widening of the tibio-fibular mortise may be overlooked unless particular note is made of the joint space at the medial side of the talus, and the difficulty of diagnosis is increased by the fact that the fibular fracture may be too high in the shaft to be seen in routine radiographs of the ankle (Fig. 16.17A). In tibio-fibular diastasis the talus is always carried laterally with the fibula, so the space between the medial malleolus and the talus is widened (Fig. 16.17A). If widening of the space is observed without a fracture of the lateral malleolus a radiograph should always be obtained of the whole length of the fibula: this will invariably show a fracture of some part of the shaft, sometimes far above the ankle (Fig. 16.17B). Even when the radiographs of the ankle region appear normal (as they may do if the displacement has been spontaneously reduced) the severe swelling and clinical disability should alert the surgeon to the need for a more extensive radiographic examination.

Treatment

Although the displacement can nearly always be reduced by manipulation it is notoriously prone to recur within the plaster despite careful moulding. For this reason operation is advised. The tibio-fibular diastasis is reduced under direct vision and the fibula is secured to the tibia by a single long screw driven transversely across the two bones (Fig. 16.17C). If the medial malleolus has been avulsed it should be fixed in position with a second screw. Post-operative management is the same as for displaced malleolar fractures (p. 287).

Posterior marginal fracture of the tibia

(Diagrams 6 and 12 in Fig. 16.12)

When the momentum of the body carries the tibia forwards upon the foot at the time of the injury the posterior articular margin of the tibia may be sheared off. Radiographs may show the talus displaced backwards upon the tibia, but sometimes a momentary displacement has been reduced spontaneously by the time the patient is seen. This posterior marginal fracture of the tibia is additional to a fracture of one or both malleoli, and it may occur in conjunction either with an abduction-rotation injury or with an adduction injury (Fig. 16.12, diagrams 6 and 12).

The separated posterior fragment of the tibia is nearly always displaced slightly upwards, forming a step in the articular surface. Fortunately the posterior fragment is usually small and the greater part of the articular surface remains intact (Fig. 16.18). Occasionally, however, the fragment includes a large area of the articular surface, and unless it is restored perfectly to position the irregular step in the surface will lead inevitably to later osteoarthritis.

Fig. 16.18 Posterior marginal fracture of the tibia with associated spiral fracture of the lateral malleolus. There is slight posterior displacement of the talus upon the tibia, as evidenced by the fact that the opposed articular surfaces of the tibia and the talus are not congruous. (This injury corresponds to that shown in Fig. 16.12, diagram 6.)

Treatment

Provided the articular surfaces of the tibia and talus are congruous, separation of a *small* posterior tibial fragment may be ignored and attention directed solely to the other components of the injury, namely the associated malleolar fracture and the displacement of the talus. However, when the posterior tibial fragment is large and includes more than a quarter of the articular surface in the lateral radiograph, it must be replaced perfectly in position. It is seldom possible to obtain a satisfactory reduction by manipulation, and in practice it is necessary to resort to operative reduction and fixation by a screw or buttress plate inserted from behind. Any associated malleolar fracture should be handled according to the principles already outlined. Thereafter the ankle is protected in plaster for 10 weeks before mobilising exercises are begun.

Vertical compression (pilon) fracture of the tibia

(Diagrams 13 and 14 in Fig. 16.12)
This injury is usually caused by a fall from a height. It is relatively uncommon, because most patients who fall from a height onto the foot sustain a fracture of the calcaneus rather than of the tibia.

A vertical force acting on the lower articular surface of the tibia may cause two types of injury, according to the severity of the violence. If the violence is only moderate, the front of the tibial articular surface is sheared off and the talus may be displaced slightly forwards (Fig. 16.12, diagram 13). If the violence is severe, there is a comminuted fracture involving the whole of the inferior articular surface of the tibia—and often also of the fibula—and the talus may be driven upwards between the two bones (Figs 16.12, diagram 14, & 16.19A).

A

B

Fig. 16.19 A Severe comminuted fracture involving the lower articular surface of the tibia. B After operative reduction and fixation by plates and screws.

Treatment

In the treatment of the less severe injuries the aim should be to secure accurate reduction of the articular fragments so that the joint surface is left perfectly smooth. This may sometimes be achieved by manipulation and immobilisation in plaster, but in most cases operative reduction and fixation by screws are required.

In the severely comminuted fractures with upward displacement of the talus it may be impossible to restore a smooth articular surface by any method. Nevertheless it is worthwhile to restore the anatomy as accurately as possible by means of cancellous bone grafts to support the articular surface, combined with appropriately placed screws or plates (Fig. 16.19B), and then to await events. If severe damage to the joint surfaces precludes the restoration of good function, arthrodesis of the ankle may be the best means of permitting painless walking.

SOFT-TISSUE INJURIES ABOUT THE ANKLE

RUPTURE OF THE LATERAL LIGAMENTS OF THE ANKLE

(Diagram 10 in Fig. 16.12)

Rarely, a severe adduction force may cause complete rupture of the talo-fibular and calcaneo-fibular ligaments, with consequent tilting and subluxation of the talus in the tibio-fibular mortise (Fig. 16.12, diagram 10).

Clinical features

There is a history of a severe adduction injury, which is followed by rapid swelling about the lateral aspect of the ankle. Later, there is extensive visible bruising. Pain is severe, so that walking is difficult or impossible.

Diagnosis

Unless the special features of this injury are recognised it may be mistaken for a simple strain of the ligaments (p. 295). The extent of the swelling and bruising, the severe pain and the marked disability should suggest the possibility of a complete tear of the ligaments even if the initial radiographs appear normal, and the diagnosis should be settled by obtaining antero-posterior radiographs while an adduction stress is applied to the heel. (An anaesthetic is necessary if the injury is recent.) If the ligaments are torn, the talus will be shown tilted medially in the tibio-fibular mortise (Fig. 16.20). A tilt of less than 20° is not necessarily abnormal: in doubtful cases the uninjured ankle should be radiographed in the same way for comparison.

Treatment

If the injury is treated as a simple strain, with early exercises and activity, the torn ligaments may fail to heal and recurrent subluxation of the ankle may ensue. If conservative treatment is to be adopted it is essential that the ligaments be protected by a below-knee plaster for not less than 8 weeks. This method is usually successful, and it is usually preferred to the alternative method of direct repair of the ligaments at operation.

Fig. 16.20 Tilting of the talus in the ankle mortise under adduction stress, an indication of torn lateral ligaments. (This injury corresponds to diagram 10 in Fig. 16.14.)

Recurrent subluxation of the ankle

When the lateral ligaments of the ankle are torn and fail to heal there may be persistent instability, with recurrent attacks of 'giving way' in which the talus tilts medially in the ankle mortise.

Clinical features

The patient complains that, after an initial injury, the ankle goes over at frequent intervals, sometimes causing a fall. Each incident is accompanied by pain at the lateral side of the ankle. *On examination* there is often some oedema about the ankle. There is tenderness over the site of the lateral ligaments. The normal ankle movements—dorsiflexion and plantarflexion—are unchanged, but abnormal mobility is present as shown by the fact that the heel can be inverted passively beyond the normal range permitted by the subtalar joint when compared with the opposite side. Moreover, when the heel is fully inverted a dimple or depression of the skin may be visible in front of the lateral malleolus, where the soft tissues have been sucked into the gap created between tibia and talus.

Radiographic examination. Routine radiographs do not show any abnormality. Antero-posterior films must be taken while the heel is held fully inverted. If the lateral ligaments are torn, the talus will be shown tilted away from the tibio-fibular mortise through 20° or more (Fig. 16.20). When the fibulo-calcaneal ligament is torn there may also be antero-posterior instability of the talus, which may glide forwards in the tibio-fibular mortise under stress.

Treatment

If the disability is slight it may be sufficient to strengthen the evertor muscles (mainly the peronei) by exercises, to enable them to control the ankle more efficiently. At the same time the heel of the shoe may be splayed laterally, or 'floated out,' to reduce the tendency to going over.

If the disability is severe operation is required. A new lateral ligament is constructed, usually by using the peroneus brevis tendon. Synthetic materials for ligament reconstruction are on trial, but their place in treatment is not yet fully established.

STRAIN OF THE LATERAL LIGAMENTS OF THE ANKLE

When adduction violence is insufficient to rupture the lateral ligaments of the ankle completely, one or more of the ligaments may be strained. (This is the common 'sprained ankle'.) Such strains are much more common than complete rupture of the ligaments. The injury corresponds to diagram 7 in Figure 16.12.

Clinical features

There are pain and swelling at the lateral aspect of the ankle, with difficulty in walking. The greatest tenderness is immediately below and in front of the lateral malleolus. There is a good range of plantarflexion and dorsiflexion at the ankle, but attempted adduction increases the pain.

Diagnosis

The possibility of a fracture must always be excluded by radiographic examination. If pain and swelling are severe, and especially if there is extensive bruising, the possibility of complete rupture of the lateral ligaments must be investigated by taking antero-posterior radiographs while an adduction stress is applied to the heel (p. 294). A lateral radiograph taken while forward pressure is applied to the foot should also be obtained, to check whether the talus is stable against anterior shift.

Treatment

In the ordinary case little or no treatment is required. The usual practice is to support the ankle for 2 weeks with a crepe bandage. If pain and swelling are unusually severe it may be wise to protect the ankle in a walking plaster for 2 or 3 weeks.

Strain of the lateral ligament of the subtalar joint

In many instances a 'sprained ankle' is in fact a strain of the lateral ligament of the subtalar (talo-calcaneal) joint rather than of the ankle joint proper. This injury is caused by excessive inversion-adduction of the foot in much the same way as a strain of the ankle ligaments, but the inversion-adduction movement is often associated with forced plantarflexion. The point of greatest tenderness is lower and further forward than in strains of the ankle ligaments, and the pain is exacerbated not so much by pure adduction as by combined adduction and plantarflexion. Treatment is the same as for strains of the ankle ligaments.

RUPTURE OF THE CALCANEAL TENDON

Surprising as it may seem, a ruptured calcaneal tendon (tendo achillis) is often overlooked, the symptoms being wrongly ascribed to a strained muscle or a ruptured plantaris tendon.

Pathology

The rupture is nearly always complete. It occurs about 5 cm above the insertion of the tendon. If it is left untreated, the tendon unites spontaneously, but with lengthening.

Fig. 16.21 The crucial test of intact calf function is to ask the patient to raise the heel from the ground while standing only on the affected leg. Inability to do this after an injury to the calcaneal tendon is diagnostic of complete rupture.

Clinical features

While running or jumping the patient feels a sudden severe pain at the back of the ankle and may believe that something has struck him. The patient is able to walk, but with a limp. *On examination* there is tenderness at the site of rupture. There is general thickening from effusion of blood and from oedema of the paratenon, but a gap can usually be felt in the course of the tendon. The power of plantarflexion at the ankle is greatly weakened, though some power remains through the action of the tibialis posterior, the peronei and the toe flexors.

Diagnosis

The retention of some power of plantarflexion may deflect the unwary from the correct diagnosis. The crucial test is to ask the patient to lift the heel from the ground while standing only upon the affected leg (Fig. 16.21). This is impossible if the tendon is ruptured. When this clinical test is equivocal, the presence of a ruptured tendon can be confirmed by the use of an ultrasound or MRI scan.

Treatment

Non-operative treatment is usually by immobilisation in a below-knee plaster case for 6 weeks, with the foot in moderate equinus to relax the tendon and thus to help to prevent lengthening. The patient should mobilise on crutches without weight-bearing for the first 2 weeks.

Operative treatment entails repair of the tendon, using either non-absorbable polypropylene or heavy braided absorbable polyglactin sutures. Tension on the suture line is relaxed by immobilising the limb with right-angled knee flexion and moderate ankle plantarflexion for 2 weeks. For the next 4 weeks a below-knee plaster with the ankle at 90° is worn. Whether treatment is by plaster alone or by operation, it must be completed after removal of the plaster by increasingly vigorous exercises for the calf muscles, practised until full strength is restored.

There is still no clear consensus on the best form of treatment for this injury. Conservative treatment is often preferred in the elderly, but carries a higher rate of re-rupture, averaging 13%. Surgical repair has only a 3% re-rupture rate and is more frequently employed for the younger athletic patient. However, it is associated with a higher risk of other complications, including wound infection and damage to the sural nerve.

Strained calf muscle

Occasionally the calf muscle is strained or 'pulled', especially during athletic pursuits. The essential pathology is probably rupture of a few muscle fibres. There is sudden severe pain, well localised in the muscular part of the calf. The pain and tenderness are considerably higher in the calf than in a case of ruptured calcaneal tendon. Moreover there is no palpable gap, and the patient is able, despite pain, to raise himself onto the toes as in Figure 16.21. These diagnostic features distinguish strain of the calf muscle from rupture of the calcaneal tendon: great care is needed in differentiating the two conditions, because failure to diagnose rupture of the calcaneal tendon may lead to persistent disability. The symptoms subside spontaneously and treatment is not required.

Rupture of the plantaris muscle

A diagnosis of rupture of the plantaris muscle must be made with caution: in many instances it has proved to be erroneous, the true condition being rupture of the calcaneal tendon itself. Rupture of the plantaris—usually near the junction of muscle and tendon—is a distinct entity, but it is very uncommon. It occurs with dramatic suddenness during running or leaping, as does rupture of the calcaneal tendon. There is sharp pain, often with later swelling and bruising. Pain and tenderness are higher in the calf than in a case of rupture of the calcaneal tendon, and a little towards the medial side, over the course of the plantaris muscle and tendon. The calcaneal tendon itself is felt to be intact, and the patient can lift the heel from the ground when standing on the affected leg (Fig. 16.21). Treatment is by firm elastic bandaging and curtailment of activities until the pain and swelling subside.

17 | The foot

CLASSIFICATION

The injuries to be described may be classified as follows:

Injuries of the tarsus

[1] Fractures and fracture-dislocations of the talus

[2] Fractures of the calcaneus

[3] Other fractures of the tarsal bones

    Mid-tarsal and tarso-metatarsal dislocations

Fractures of the metatarsal bones and phalanges of the toes

[4] Fractures of the metatarsal bones

[5] Fractures of the phalanges of the toes

The foot

In contrast to injuries of the ankle, injuries of the foot are surprisingly uncommon. Among the more frequent of those that occur are fractures of the calcaneus from falls onto the heels, which often lead to residual disability, and fractures of the metatarsals and phalanges of the toes, which are usually benign.

INJURIES OF THE TARSUS

FRACTURES OF THE TALUS

In most injuries caused by a fall from a height onto the feet it is the calcaneus that gives way under the stress, and fractures of the talus are uncommon. Most serious fractures of the talus occur through the neck of the bone, but minor fractures are also encountered in which a small chip or flake is detached, usually from the margin of one of the articular surfaces.

Fracture of the neck of the talus

This major fracture was once termed 'aviator's astragalus' because of its frequent occurrence in the pilots of crashed aircraft, when the rudder-bar was driven forcibly up against the middle of the sole of the foot. In peacetime the injury occurs far more commonly in the drivers of vehicles involved in road traffic accidents, when the foot pedals can cause a similar mechanism of injury. The impact forces the forefoot and the head of the talus upwards and the bone fractures through the neck of the talus as it is driven against the inferior margin of the tibia (Fig. 17.1A). The fracture may be relatively undisplaced, but in more severe injuries the body of the talus may be dislocated backwards out of the ankle mortise (Fig. 17.1B). When displacement or dislocation occurs, damage to

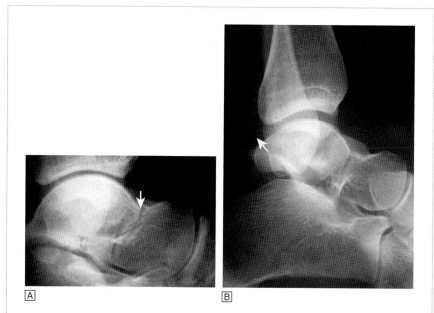

Fig. 17.1 A Lateral radiograph showing fracture of the neck of the talus (arrow). B Fracture-dislocation of the talus with posterior displacement of body (arrow).

the major nutrient artery to the body of the talus is inevitable and the incidence of subsequent avascular necrosis is high.

Treatment

In undisplaced fractures through the neck of the talus immobilisation in a below-knee plaster cast for 10–12 weeks is the appropriate treatment, though the blood supply to the body of the talus should be monitored at intervals. In displaced fractures or fracture-dislocations an open reduction is usually required to ensure exact apposition of the fragments prior to internal fixation with cannulated cancellous screws. Thereafter the ankle is protected in a below-knee plaster, often for 10–12 weeks, to provide the best conditions for union. Weight-bearing on the affected foot should be avoided for at least the first 6 weeks, but walking with crutches is permitted.

Complications

Non-union and avascular necrosis. Fractures through the neck of the talus are prone to non-union, which is often associated with avascular necrosis of the proximal (body) fragment from damage to the nutrient vessels at the time of the injury. In its tendency to develop avascular changes the fractured talus closely resembles the fractured scaphoid bone in the wrist. The effects are similar as the avascular fragment often fails to unite with the rest of the bone, it gradually collapses, and the overlying articular cartilage is shed.

Diagnosis. As in the scaphoid bone, avascular necrosis of the talus may be recognised 1 or 2 months after the injury by a marked difference in the radiographic density of the affected fragment compared with the surrounding bones. The avascular bone does not share in the osteoporosis that occurs from disuse in the foot as a whole; so it appears much denser than the neighbouring bones. Diagnosis may also be aided by MRI scanning. In the later stages the diagnosis is obvious because the affected bone collapses into an amorphous mass.

Treatment. If the fracture fails to unite and avascular necrosis is recognised, operation is required. The aim should be to eliminate the peri-talar joints (the ankle, subtalar and talo-navicular joints) by arthrodesis. If avascular necrosis has led to marked collapse and disintegration of the body of the talus, it may be necessary to excise the avascular remnants and to fuse the tibia to the upper surface of the calcaneus.

Osteoarthritis. Osteoarthritis of the ankle and subtalar joints is almost inevitable after avascular necrosis of the body of the talus. Arthritis may also follow injury to the articular surface without avascular necrosis. If arthritis becomes disabling, the only satisfactory treatment is to eliminate the affected joint or joints by arthrodesis.

Minor fractures of the talus

Minor fractures in which a small chip or flake of bone is pulled off the talus are more common than the serious fractures just described. They often accompany severe strains of the ankle and occur at the site of ligamentous insertions. There is seldom severe displacement, though the fractures may be frequently missed and present later with recurrent pain and instability of the ankle.

Fig. 17.2 Osteochondral fracture from the articular surface of the dome of the talus (arrow).

Less commonly a severe shearing injury to the dome of the talus may result in detachment of a larger osteochondral fragment (Fig. 17.2). Treatment depends on the size of the fragment; when large it can be replaced in its bed with a Herbert type screw, but smaller fragments should be removed arthroscopically or by open arthrotomy with drilling of the defect to encourage healing.

FRACTURES OF THE CALCANEUS

A fracture of the calcaneus may take the form of an isolated crack or minor fracture without displacement—usually in the region of the tuberosity—or of a compression injury which crushes the bone from above downwards. The more serious compression type of injury is unfortunately the more common.

Mechanism of injury

Almost all fractures of the calcaneus are caused by a fall from a height onto the heels: thus both heels may be injured at the same time. The type of fracture depends mainly upon the severity of the force, and therefore to a large extent on the height of the fall. The weight thrust is transmitted through the talus to the upper articular surface of the calcaneus. If this surface holds, the force is transmitted through the bone towards the tuberosity, which may be split or cracked. More usually, however, the articular surface of the calcaneus fails to withstand the stress: it is shattered by the impact and driven downwards into the body of the bone, crushing the delicate trabeculae of cancellous bone into powder. In addition, fractures radiate from the subtalar region into the tuberosity, and often also to the front of the calcaneus, emerging at the surface of the calcaneo-cuboid joint.

Minor fracture without compression

Clinical features

There is a history of a fall onto the heel, not usually from more than a few feet. There is severe local pain, and the patient is unable to put weight on the heel. Examination reveals a little soft-tissue swelling about the heel, marked local tenderness over the tuberosity of the calcaneus, but no palpable deformity of the bone. Later, an ecchymosis may be observed in the sole of the foot at the sides of the plantar aponeurosis. Movements of the ankle, subtalar and mid-tarsal joints are not appreciably restricted.

Fig. 17.3 Ⓐ Isolated fracture of tuberosity of the calcaneus without displacement. The fracture is seen best in the axial radiograph Ⓑ. The subtalar joint surface is intact. Note the normal shape of the calcaneus, for comparison with that of the crushed calcaneus shown in Figure 17.5.

Diagnosis

The fracture may be overlooked unless adequate radiographic examination is carried out. It is not sufficient to rely only upon the ordinary lateral projection of the heel, which may fail to show the fracture. An axial view is essential: the central ray is projected obliquely through the heel from the plantar surface while the ankle is held fully dorsiflexed (Fig. 17.3B).

Treatment

Unlike the more serious compression fractures, isolated fractures of the calcaneus without displacement present little difficulty in treatment. All that is required is to protect the heel for 4 weeks or so by a below-knee plaster (see Fig. 16.13), in which walking may be allowed almost from the beginning. Excellent results may be expected, and complications are exceptional.

Compression fracture

A compression fracture of the calcaneus must be regarded as a serious injury which leads inevitably to permanent impairment of function despite the most careful treatment.

Clinical features

There is a history of a fall onto the heels, often from a considerable height. Both heels may be injured together. The patient is unable to bear weight on the affected foot or feet. On examination, the heel is palpably broadened out sideways, and careful measurements taken from the malleoli to the under surface of the heel may show that it is reduced in height. There is marked local tenderness over the calcaneus. After 1 or 2 days a visible ecchymosis spreads into the sole of the foot at the sides of the plantar aponeurosis—a characteristic

Fig. 17.4 Characteristic distribution of the visible bruising from a fracture of the calcaneus. The tough central part of the plantar aponeurosis forms a barrier, preventing spread of the ecchymosis to the weight-bearing part of the sole. Discolouration therefore spreads towards the sides of the heel and the medial aspect of the instep.

feature (Fig. 17.4). Movements of the ankle are not appreciably impaired, but there is marked restriction of inversion—eversion movement at the subtalar and midtarsal joints, which are nearly always damaged.

In many cases of crush fracture of the calcaneus there is also a compression fracture of a vertebral body, usually in the lower thoracic or upper lumbar region. This common association is explained by the fact that the two fractures are caused by the same type of injury, namely a fall from a height.

Diagnosis

Unlike a minor crack fracture, a compression fracture of the calcaneus is easily diagnosed from the lateral radiograph if the shape of the bone is compared with the normal (Figs 17.3 & 17.5). The most striking feature is that the upper surface of the calcaneus is distinctly flattened, so that the line of the subtalar joint may form almost a straight line with the upper surface of the tuberosity. This 'tuberosity-joint angle' (normally about 35–40°) has been used as an index of the severity of the compression: in a severe case the angle is reduced to zero or it may even be inverted. The introduction of CT scanning has allowed far more accurate visualisation of the fracture configuration and the extent of subtalar joint involvement (Fig.17.6). It has also facilitated planning of surgical reduction and fixation in selected cases.

Treatment

Many different methods of treatment have been advocated for this difficult fracture, but it has to be admitted, that only very seldom is the foot restored to anything resembling normal. Some permanent disability usually has to be accepted. The main difficulty arises from the fact that the articular facets of the subtalar joint may be shattered into numerous fragments, which are driven

The foot

Fig. 17.5 Compression fracture of the calcaneus. The subtalar joint surface, especially its posterior part, has been crushed down into the body of the bone. This is indicated by the flattened outline of the upper surface of the bone (compare with the normal contour seen in Fig. 17.3). The fracture line also enters the calcaneo-cuboid joint.

Fig. 17.6 Ⓐ Axial and Ⓑ sagittal CT scans of compression fracture into the body of the calcaneus with disruption of the subtalar joint.

down into the underlying cancellous bone. Thus it is almost impossible both to restore the general shape of the bone and to refashion a perfectly smooth articular surface.

Despite these difficulties, there has been an increasing trend in recent years towards the adoption of a more aggressive policy than that which prevailed in the past, with the aim of securing accurate reduction of the displaced fragments, preferably at open operation, or by a semi-closed manoeuvre using leverage from behind by a Steinmann pin.

Open reduction and internal fixation. Techniques of open reduction have been facilitated since the introduction of CT scanning, by which the geography of the complex fracture may be precisely demonstrated. The calcaneus is exposed from the lateral side, and after the main fragments have been levered back to their normal location the position is held by packing with cancellous bone grafts and the application of plates and screws. This should now be regarded as the preferred method of treatment when conditions are favourable.

Reduction by closed leverage. When the calcaneal tuberosity is displaced markedly upwards it is possible, after driving a stout Steinmann pin into the bone from behind, to lever the tuberosity downwards to restore the bone approximately to its former shape. When the best possible reduction has been gained, the foot is encased in a plaster-of-Paris slipper with the percutaneous pin incorporated in the plaster. The foot should be elevated for long periods to reduce swelling, but a little walking with crutches may be allowed. After removal of the plaster, intensive exercises are practised under the supervision of a physiotherapist to restore as much mobility as the inevitable adhesions will allow.

Conservative treatment. Conservative treatment was for many years the mainstay in the management of calcaneal fractures. The principles of conservative treatment are to accept the displacement, to avoid immobilisation, and to encourage movement of the joints from the beginning. It is hoped that in this way the pliable granulations that form over the shattered joint surfaces in the process of healing will be moulded to a reasonably smooth contour and that intra-articular adhesions will be minimised. To this end the foot is elevated to reduce oedema. Active exercises are begun at once to encourage movement at the ankle, subtalar and midtarsal joints. Ankle movement (plantarflexion/dorsiflexion) is usually regained without difficulty because the joint surfaces are undamaged, but there is always considerable restriction of subtalar and midtarsal movement (inversion/eversion), which yields gradually, though incompletely, to intensive exercises.

Complications

Stiffness of the subtalar and midtarsal joints. Some impairment of inversion-eversion movement is an almost inevitable sequel of a compression fracture of the calcaneus, because the subtalar joint (and often also the midtarsal joint) is nearly always extensively damaged. Though stiffness cannot be prevented altogether, it can be kept to a minimum by insisting upon elevation of the foot for several weeks after the injury to control oedema, and by encouraging early active exercises.

Osteoarthritis. The subtalar joint is often left distorted and irregular after a compression fracture of the calcaneus, and osteoarthritis is a common sequel; indeed, the surprising fact is that it does not always become disabling. In some cases severe pain does cause serious disability at an early stage, and demands operative treatment; but in others the patient may be able to carry on indefinitely with only slight pain and with little disability. The symptoms are always aggravated by walking on rough ground.

Treatment. It is probable that the development of severe osteoarthritis may, to some extent, be prevented by mobilising exercises begun soon after the injury. When established arthritis becomes disabling the only satisfactory treatment is by arthrodesis of the subtalar joint and, if necessary, of the midtarsal joint.

Limp. An effect of severe depression of the subtalar articular surface is that the calcaneal tuberosity—and with it the insertion of the calcaneal tendon—is displaced proximally. In consequence, the calf muscles are unduly slack, and the power of raising the heel from the ground is impaired. This loss of 'spring' may cause a persistent slight limp, and it is a feature that may argue in support of those who favour operative reduction of the deformity in the first instance. Treatment is by intensive exercises for the calf muscles, which may be able, eventually, to take up the slack.

Associated fracture of the spine. The frequent association between crush fracture of the calcaneus and compression fracture of a vertebral body has already been mentioned. The spinal column should be examined clinically and radiographically in every case of calcaneal fracture, whether or not there are any symptoms in the spine. Only thus can the risk of overlooking a spinal fracture be avoided.

OTHER INJURIES OF THE TARSAL BONES

Fractures of the other tarsal bones are uncommon, and do not require detailed consideration here. Dislocation of the tarsal joints is also uncommon. It may occur at the subtalar joint, at the midtarsal joint (Fig. 17.7) or at the tarso-metatarsal joints, and at any of these sites dislocation may be associated with a fracture. The principles of treatment are to reduce the dislocation and thereafter

Fig. 17.7 Mid-tarsal dislocation of the foot (arrow).

Fig. 17.8 Tarso-metatarsal fracture-subluxation. Note the fracture of the base of the third metatarsal, with lateral displacement of the outer three metatarsals.

to immobilise the foot in a below-knee walking plaster for 6 or 8 weeks. When manipulative reduction is impossible, operation may be required, and if the joint is badly shattered arthrodesis may have to be considered.

Mid-tarsal dislocation

These uncommon injuries are usually caused by a severe adduction or abduction force applied to the forefoot from a motor vehicle or sporting injury. Radiographs often show an associated avulsion fracture at the site of dislocation in the talo-navicular and calcaneo-cuboid joints (Fig. 17.7). The injury is frequently associated with marked soft-tissue swelling, or even circulatory impairment, making early reduction essential. This can usually be achieved by closed manipulation under anaesthesia, but additional stabilisation with percutaneous Kirschner wires may be required to prevent redisplacement. The limb should then be immobilised in a non-weight-bearing below-knee plaster cast for 6 weeks. The main complication of this injury is the risk of the later onset of secondary osteoarthritis.

Tarso-metartarsal dislocation

Dislocation or subluxation at the tarso-metatarsal joints (Lisfranc's fracture-dislocation[1]) is uncommon. It is usually caused by forced inversion or eversion of the forefoot when the hindfoot is fixed, or occasionally by a crushing injury

---

[1] Jacques Lisfranc was a field surgeon with Napoleon's army on the Russian front. He did not describe the fracture dislocation, but in 1815 described the amputation through the tarso-metatarsal joints which bears his name.

The foot

of the foot. Soft-tissue swelling often masks the bony deformity and makes clinical diagnosis difficult. Radiological diagnosis (Fig. 17.8) may also be difficult, especially if partial reduction of the displacement has occurred.

The principles of treatment are to reduce the dislocation and thereafter to immobilise the foot in a below-knee walking plaster for 6–8 weeks. If manipulative reduction is impossible, operation may be required: after reposition of the parts in anatomical relationship, the position may be stabilised by the insertion across the joints of thin stiff (Kirschner) wires, which may be removed 6 or 8 weeks later. If the joint is badly shattered (comminuted fracture-dislocation), satisfactory reconstruction may be impracticable and arthrodesis may have to be considered.

FRACTURES OF THE METATARSAL BONES AND PHALANGES OF THE TOES

FRACTURES OF THE METATARSAL BONES

Most metatarsal fractures are caused by direct violence from a heavy object falling on the foot. A metatarsal may also be fractured by muscular violence in a twisting injury, or by repeated stress without any specific injury (stress or fatigue fractures).

Fracture of the base of the fifth metatarsal

Fracture of the base of the fifth metatarsal bone is common. It is nearly always caused by a twisting injury in which the foot is forced into inversion and equinus. It is an avulsion fracture, the styloid process at the base of the metatarsal being pulled off by the tendon of the peroneus brevis muscle, which is inserted into it.

Clinically, there is pain at the outer border of the foot, with difficulty in walking. There is marked local tenderness over the base of the metatarsal, and the diagnosis of fracture is easily confirmed by radiography (Fig. 17.9A).

A less common, but more serious, injury is the Jones[2] fracture at the base of the 5th metatarsal. It results from local trauma to the lateral side of the foot producing a transverse fracture through the junction of the metaphysis and shaft (Fig. 17.9B). It is more common in footballers and other professional athletes, and in a few patients may represent a chronic fatigue fracture.

Treatment

Although immobilisation is not essential to union of the fracture, a plaster should usually be advised for the relief of pain. A below-knee walking plaster of standard type (see Fig. 16.13) is used. The plaster need not be retained for longer than 3 weeks, and thereafter the only treatment required is a course of active exercise to restore movement and muscle tone. In younger athletes or where there is delayed union it may be necessary to undertake internal fixation of the fracture with a cancellous screw.

---

[2] Sir Robert Jones, the father of British orthopaedic surgery, described this fracture in his own foot in 1902 when he sustained the injury while dancing around a Maypole at a Garden Party.

Fig. 17.9 A Avulsion fracture of the base of the fifth metatarsal bone caused by forcible inversion of the foot (arrow). B Jones fracture of metaphysis at the base of the fifth metatarsal (arrow).

Os vesalianum

In childhood the single epiphysis of the fifth metatarsal is normally at the distal end, as it is also in the second, third and fourth metatarsals. Occasionally, an accessory ossicle, the os vesalianum, is seen in relation to the base of the fifth metatarsal, and it may be mistaken for a fragment avulsed from the base of the metatarsal by injury. Differentiation is aided by the fact that these accessory ossicles are nearly always bilateral and, in case of doubt, the uninjured foot should be radiographed for comparison.

Fractures of the metatarsal shafts

One or more of the metatarsals may be fractured by a heavy object falling on the foot. The fracture may occur at any point in the shaft: near the base, in the mid-shaft, or at the metatarsal neck. It is usually of the transverse or short oblique type, and displacement is seldom severe (Fig. 17.10).

Treatment

Here again immobilisation is required mainly for the relief of pain: union will occur readily whether or not the fracture is immobilised. As a rule a walking plaster should be worn for 3 or 4 weeks and, thereafter, active exercises should be arranged.

Fig. 17.10 Fractures of the second and third metatarsal bones from a crushing injury.

Fatigue or stress fracture of a metatarsal bone ('March' fracture)

The general subject of fatigue or stress fracture was considered in Chapter 1, page 14. Fatigue fractures occur more commonly in the metatarsals than in any other bone. They differ from ordinary fractures in that there is no history of violence: the pain seems to arise spontaneously and the possibility of a fracture may be overlooked.

Cause

The fracture is ascribed to long-continued or oft-repeated stress, particularly from prolonged walking or running, in those who are not accustomed to it. Thus, it may occur in army recruits freshly committed to marching; hence the term 'march fracture'. It has been likened to the fatigue fractures that sometimes occur in metals.

Pathology

The fracture usually affects the shaft or neck of the second or third metatarsal bone. It is no more than a hair-line crack, and there is no displacement of the fragments. In the process of healing a large mass of callus may form around the bone at the site of fracture.

Clinical features

The complaint is of severe pain in the forefoot on walking. The onset is rapid but the patient is usually unable to ascribe it to an obvious cause. Enquiry may reveal, however, that there has been an unusual amount of walking 1 or 2 days before the onset. Indeed, the pain often begins during a march. On examination there is swelling on the dorsum of the foot, with well marked local tenderness

| A | | B |

Fig. 17.11 A typical march or fatigue fracture of the second metatarsal. In the initial radiograph Ⓐ, taken soon after the onset of symptoms, the fracture is seen only as a faint hair-line crack. Ⓑ Two weeks later the fracture is surrounded by abundant callus.

over the affected metatarsal. Radiographs at first show only a faint hair-line crack which may be easily overlooked (Fig. 17.11A), but after 1 or 2 weeks the callus surrounding the fracture is clearly visible (Fig. 17.11B).

Treatment
The fracture heals spontaneously, so treatment is purely symptomatic. In some cases no treatment is needed, but if pain is severe, immobilisation in a below-knee walking plaster for 4 weeks is advised.

FRACTURES OF THE PHALANGES OF THE TOES

Most fractures of the toes are caused by crushing injuries, as from the fall of a heavy object. The great toe, being the most prominent, is the one most often affected. In many cases the phalanx is severely comminuted, but a satisfactory general alignment is preserved. Sometimes the fracture is associated with a bursting wound of the skin and soft tissues. Swelling and pain are often severe.

Treatment
Little or no treatment is required for these fractures. If there is much swelling, with severe pain, it is wise to elevate the foot for a few days, but otherwise the only treatment required is to protect the toe from accidental knocks by a soft woolly dressing.

Further reading

Detailed references on individual fractures and their management have been omitted from this edition of *Outline of Fractures* since they rapidly become out of date and are not required by the average reader of an introductory text. For those who are stimulated to seek more information on the specialised treatment of musculoskeletal injuries we have listed the most commonly used advanced textbooks in the field, most of which are now available in both print and digital format.

We also thought it would be helpful to provide a short reading list of key historical books and references that have influenced the developments in fracture care and the understanding of their pathology and healing mechanisms. This list is not intended as a comprehensive guide even to the more recent literature on fracture surgery: space does not permit the inclusion of more than a limited selection. Many of the texts are now out of print, but should still be available in larger medical libraries. An original description or a classic paper has not always been listed when reference to it is made in more recent works, because it can thereby be easily traced. In the main, the references are to works in the English language, which will be readily accessible to most readers.

Titles printed in *italics* refer to books or monographs: those printed in roman type refer to papers in journals.

ADVANCED TEXTBOOKS OF FRACTURE MANAGEMENT

Rockwood and Green's Fractures in Adults, 6th ed., edit Bucholz, R.W., et al. (2005): Lippincott Williams & Wilkins.
(The most widely used and comprehensive standard reference text for the detailed management of fractures and joint injuries in adults.)
Wenger, D.R., Pring, M.E. & Rang, M. (2005): *Rang's Children's Fractures,* (3rd ed). Lippincott Williams & Wilkins.
(A well established text dealing with the management of musculoskeletal injuries in children.)
Heim, U., Mueller, M.E., Nazarian, S., Koch, P., & Schatzker, J. (1994): *The Comprehensive Classification of Fractures of Long Bones,* Berlin: Springer–Verlag.
(Describes the detailed method of the AO classification for all long bone fractures, which has been widely adopted as the standard in most trauma services.)

HISTORICAL TEXTS IN THE EVOLUTION OF FRACTURE CARE

Watson-Jones, R. (1955): *Fractures and Joint Injuries,* 4th ed., Edinburgh: E. & S. Livingstone.
(First published in 1940 and Regarded by many as the 'Bible' for the care of musculoskeletal injuries, running into several editions and translated into many languages.)
Charnley, J. (1970): *The Closed Treatment of Common Fractures,* (3rd ed.). Edinburgh: Churchill Livingston.

Further reading

(Probably the best account of the principles of using manipulation and traction for the reduction and immobilisation of limb fractures.)

Mears, D.C. (1983): *External Skeletal Fixation.* Baltimore: Williams & Wilkins.

(A comprehensive coverage of the historical development of all types of external fixation and their application to a wide range of open and closed fractures.)

Stewart, J.D.M., & Hallet, J.P. (1983): *Traction and Orthopaedic Appliances.* Edinburgh: Churchill Livingston.

(Provides a detailed account of the wide range of traction and splintage techniques popular in the era prior to the more widespread adoption of internal fixation for limb fractures.)

Sarmiento, A. & Latta, L.L. (1995): *Functional Fracture Bracing,* Berlin: Springer–Verlag.

(Describes the methods and results of functional cast bracing for diaphyseal fractures of the tibia, humerus and ulna.)

Müller, M.E., Allgöwer, M., Schneider, R., & Willenegger, H. (1991): *Manual of Internal Fixation* (3rd ed.). Berlin: Springer-Verlag.

(Describes the techniques recommended by the originators of the AO system for the compression fixation of fractures and the mechanical principles underlying the system.)

Schatzker, J. & Tile, M. (1996) *The Rationale of Operative Fracture Care* (2nd ed.). Berlin: Springer–Verlag.

(Written by two exponents of the AO system describing the surgical indications, as well as the techniques for its use, for the operative care of fractures by internal fixation.)

Ham, A.W., & Harris, W.R. (1956): *Repair and transplantation of bone.* In The Biochemistry and Physiology of Bone (ed. Bourne). New York:Academic Press.

(A classic illustrated description of fracture healing that has been the basis of most subsequent research on the subject).

Trueta, J. (1963): *The role of the vessels in osteogenesis.* Journal of Bone and Joint Surgery. 45B, 402.

(One of a series of scientific papers from this famous surgeon scientist describing the role of blood vessels in bone development and healing).

Index